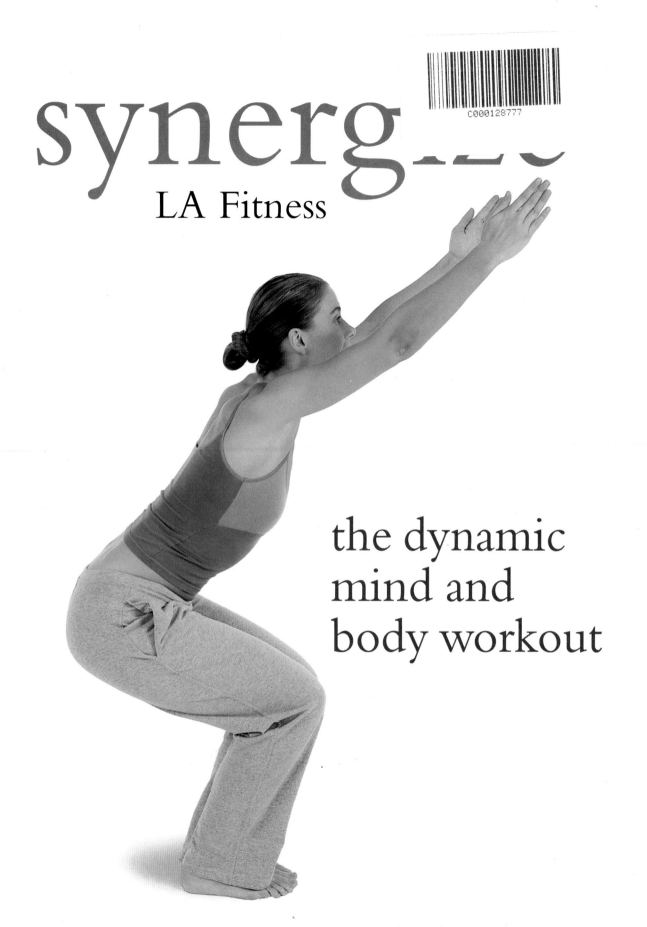

synergize

LA Fitness

the dynamic
mind and
body workout

LA Fitness is the trading name of
LA Leisure Ltd

First published in Great Britain in 2003
by Hamlyn, a division of Octopus
Publishing Group Ltd
2-4 Heron Quays, London
E14 4JP

ISBN 0 600 60623 6

A CIP catalogue record for this book is
available from the British Library

Printed and bound in China

10 9 8 7 6 5 4 3 2 1

It is advisable to check with your doctor
before embarking on any exercise
programme. Synergize™ should not be
considered a replacement for professional
medical treatment; a physician should be
consulted in all matters related to health
and particularly in respect of pregnancy
and any symptoms which may require
diagnosis or medical attention. While the
advice given in this book is believed to
be accurate and the step-by-step
instructions have been devised to avoid
strain, neither the author nor publisher
can accept any legal responsibility for
any injury sustained while following the
exercises. Please note that before using
essential oils, it is strongly recommended
that you seek advice from a doctor,
pharmacist or qualified aromatherapist.

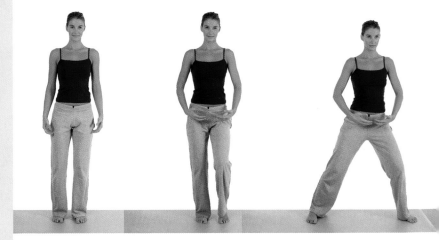

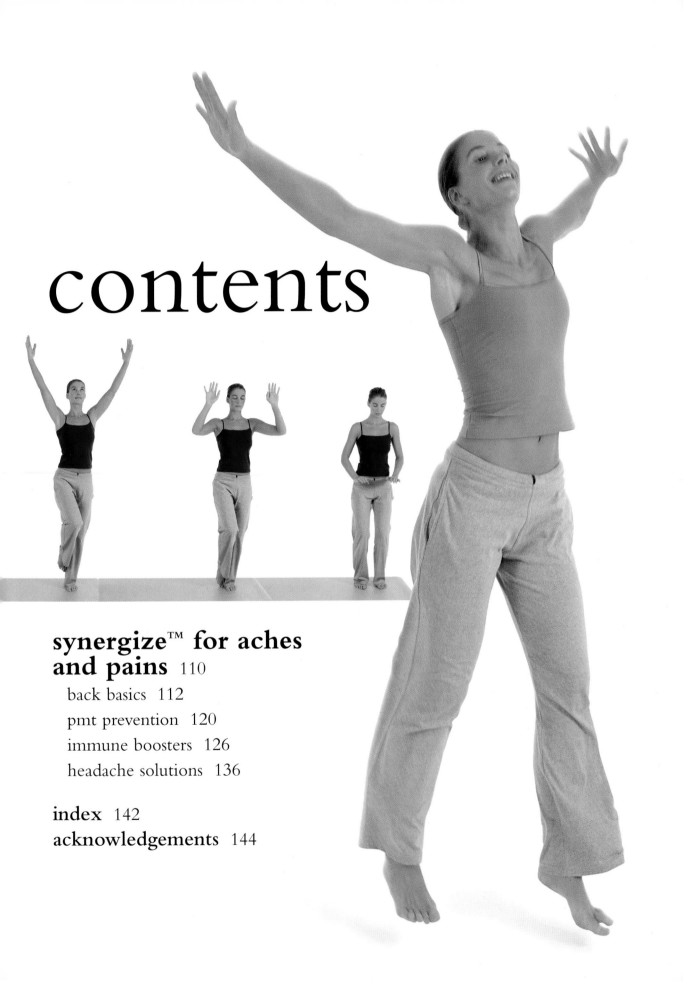

contents

foreword

Award-winning UK health club operator, LA Fitness, is one of the market innovators when it comes to offering a wide range of fitness options in a convenient location. With the aim of being the friendliest club in town and providing health and fitness in a fun, vibrant environment, it is not surprising that thousands of people across the UK choose to workout in an LA Fitness club. Now established as one of Britain's fastest growing and most successful health club operators, LA Fitness has entered the European market and expansion plans are set to continue both at home and abroad.

Each club has a modern studio that hosts an extensive range of traditional and innovative new classes. While classic classes such as aerobics and step are still taught, interest is growing in the more holistic teachings of Eastern origin such as yoga and Tai Chi. LA Fitness recognized the need to provide members with more mind and body exercises and, as a result, has developed one of the most comprehensive Mind and Body fusion programmes available in the UK today.

Extensive research by LA Fitness and spearheaded by one of their highly acclaimed experts, Jacqueline Lysycia, who specializes in dance, yoga and Pilates-based movement, involved the consultation of highly committed experts in Chi Kung, yoga, ballet and Pilates. The potential for huge benefits to be gained from merging together, in one class, the principles of traditional teachings and more modern Western disciplines was identified. The outcome was Synergize™.

A Synergize™ class combines Eastern disciplines such as yoga and Tai Chi with Western elements of core stability and body sculpting. The results have been amazing. As well as helping to produce a leaner, more toned body with improved flexibility it can also provide stress relief and improved concentration - the ideal way to feel fitter in both body and mind. Some members have seen improved body shape after following a daily fifteen minute routine.

All ages and abilities can reap the reward of regular Synergize™ sessions. The moves are uncomplicated, with fluid motion requiring no intense physical exertion. In some cases, even those recovering from injury can benefit from the improved joint flexibility and range of movement Synergize™ promotes.

At LA Fitness, Synergize™ is delivered by a team of highly trained, committed professionals, with a strong and respected background in teaching. Continuous training ensures that all teachers are knowledgeable in the latest findings and that the classes are continuously evolving to include new concepts from both the East and the West.

Synergize™ is unique to LA Fitness. The teachings in this book will provide a basic introduction and allow you to enjoy the benefits of Synergize™ from the comfort of your own home. If the book whets your appetite and you would like to learn more about Synergize™ please contact LA Fitness on (+44) 800 358 6030.

basics for life

synergy, *n*
the working together of two
or more forces to produce an
effect greater than the sum
of their individual effects.

}

Synergize™ is a powerful energy-enhancing programme developed by leading experts, health club operator LA Fitness, after extensive scientific research in the UK, Australia and India.

It produces a deep vitality that will improve every aspect of your life. A dynamic fusion of principles from Eastern and Western disciplines, **Synergize**™ combines up-to-date research and modern movement patterns with ancient philosophies. The five elements that are fused together for optimal results are:

yoga
The union of body and mind to stretch and lengthen the body.

chi kung
Breathing and meditation to cope with emotional stress and restore the nervous system to a serene and balanced state.

pilates
Movement principles that strengthen the back and abdominals from the inside out.

strength training
Creating toned and conditioned muscles for daily and functional strength.

ballet
Extension movements to lengthen and sculpt the muscles.

what is synergize™ and why do it?

The stresses we now encounter on a daily basis are very different from those of even just ten years ago and the ways in which we can choose to stay healthy in both mind and body should reflect this lifestyle change. Jumping around in an aerobics class or pounding on the treadmill are not conducive to good health if your energy is depleted by other aspects of your lifestyle, and it can make exercise a constant hardship. If you always feel lethargic, heavy and tired or you want to improve your shape but are too busy or drained by your day to exercise, then Synergize™ could be just what you are looking for.

synergize™ and the power of the mind

If you have ever tried to lose weight or start an exercise programme and failed, you were probably just focusing on your body and not your mind. Wellbeing is radiated from your inner self to the outer cells and the only way to achieve success in becoming slimmer, stronger, fitter and healthier is to get your mind and body to work together. Your mind alone is more powerful than your body. The mind is the driver, your body the vehicle. Your mind decides where you want to go and how fast you will get there, and will determine your mood and level of motivation.

By fusing the power of the motivated mind with principles from yoga, Chi Kung, Pilates, ballet and traditional strength training, Synergize™ covers all aspects of wellbeing and provides you with the optimum performance to help you cope with the stress of modern living.

how does synergize™ work?

Synergize™ teaches you how to be aware of the relationship between your inner (mind) and outer (body) self. Through the very act of exercising –

your mind and your body – you are making significant positive achievements mentally, which in turn benefits the physical body systems so that they function better, producing a feeling of inner radiance and energy. The fact that you will become leaner, stronger, fitter and healthier are all additional positive outcomes of the 'feel good' factor.

the need for synergize™

Modern lifestyles tend to involve lots of sitting, which in turn tightens muscle groups and can change the natural shape of our spines. We commonly work longer hours than ever before, and tend to play harder and eat, smoke or drink a little more to compensate for mental stress. Most of us lead very busy lives, juggling family, home, work and children. This in turn creates cluttered, fast-moving minds and we sometimes find it hard to focus mentally and to fit routine exercise and wellbeing into our daily lives on a long-term basis.

The Synergize™ programme has successfully addressed all of these issues of modern living for thousands of people – classes are now run at most LA Fitness clubs – and it can do the same for you with as little as 15 minutes' practice per day.

who is synergize™ for?

To feel good is to look good. Synergize™ has such a varied multi-dimensional format that thousands of men and women have already experienced significant benefits while working with the programme. Anyone, regardless of time or pressure constraints, age and occupation or lifestyle limitations, can enhance their way of living and energy stores. Synergize™ will produce a deep vitality that will improve every aspect of your life.

anyone can synergize™

Designed to be performed in as little as 15 minutes per day, the Synergize™ programme can fit into any lifestyle. It will help you to perform well in your specific circumstances, if you are at home, your workplace or on the move, rather than just feeling that you are making progress on the weights machines at the gym.

Essentially, the programme is for anyone who wants to enhance their energy output for functional everyday life. Whether you are a student, pensioner, housewife, office-, shop- or factory-worker, manager or director, whether you work full- or part-time or not at all, the programme suits all ages, fitness levels and abilities. Anyone interested in becoming stronger, longer, leaner and more flexible for life from the inside out will benefit from this intelligent training system for the mind and body.

The Synergize™ programme is ideal for newcomers to exercise as it is easy to follow,

MIND STRETCH

It is no coincidence that when you feel good you actually look pretty good, too. Your outer shell is an indicator of how you feel inside, which is why Synergize™ will teach you how to harness the power of your amazing synergetic mind to work in harmony with your body, to *feel* and consequently *look* better.

'If you stimulate your mind you will benefit your body. If you stimulate your body you will benefit your mind.'

teaches correct body awareness and increases muscular strength, balance and flexibility with no impact, jarring movements or intense physical exertion, which tend to work against the body's natural defence mechanisms. It is also the perfect programme for fitter pupils looking for deeper level exercises which really absorb the mind and body beyond levels currently achieved, to complement existing training programmes on a daily basis.

Synergize™ is realistic about life in the 21st century and will help you understand that mind and body wellbeing can make a small change to every single day of your life from now on.

practice gets results

Your success with the programme will inevitably depend on your own unique medical background, energy levels and personal feelings encountered when undertaking any Synergize™ movement. Although practising by yourself will bring about enormous benefits, having access to a teacher (available at most LA Fitness health clubs) will help correct your alignment and make sure that you are moving into the postures correctly. But, like learning to swim, the real journey begins when you go out into the ocean by yourself and cultivate your own energy from the programme. Make Synergize™ your own, learn from the inside, noticing any sensations in your body as you practise. Synergize™ aims to transfer the intelligence of your mind to your body through practising, listening to your body and breathing.

the elements of
synergize™

Synergize™ combines the essential mind and body elements necessary for the total unification of energy and life. It fuses the proven successful principles of Eastern holistic healing with the equally successful elements of Westernized postural, core stability and strength exercises. The main principles are concerned with the mind as well as the physical benefits of flexibility (yoga), improved breathing (Chi Kung), postural realignment and body awareness (Pilates), and improved strength and muscle tone (strength training and ballet).

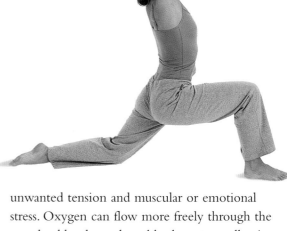

yoga

Flexibility is a basic need and is reflected within the stretch reflex reaction of a yawn and the basic desire to stretch after getting up after a long sleep or after being in a cramped position for a long period of time. Yoga, which means union, is excellent for achieving a good level of physical flexibility and also ensures that the mind and body are unified via the synergy of breath, body, mind and spirit to achieve true mental and physical flexibility.

A yogic salutation is a powerful combination of age-old movements from Hindu philosophy adapted to recharge your energy and balance your bones, muscles and bodily systems. Synergize™ uses yoga poses in between the Life Salutation (see pages 44–109) combinations to lengthen muscles and to strengthen your mind and body together as one.

When your body is flexible and strong, your joints are able to move freely within a full range of motion, making movement efficient, enjoyable and injury free. When your mind and body are calm, balanced and in perfect synergy your whole nervous system functions more smoothly, sending the correct messages to your muscles to release unwanted tension and muscular or emotional stress. Oxygen can flow more freely through the muscles, blood vessels and body systems allowing your body to be more open for change.

chi kung

A discipline linked with traditional Chinese medicine, Chi Kung is a means of cultivating energy by training the breath with slow conscious movements. Synergize™ uses breathing exercises developed from Chi Kung movements to balance the more dynamic exercise combinations outlined in the programme.

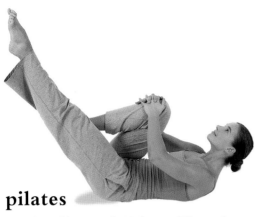

'It's not what you do,
it is the way that you do it.'
Joseph Hubertus Pilates

pilates

Developed by Joseph Hubertus Pilates, the movement principles of Pilates are successful in improving health, postural realignment, circulation and the immune system.

Born in 1880 in Dusseldorf, Joseph Pilates was a frail and sickly child. He was determined to overcome his fragility and instead of following established fitness regimes of the time he experimented with many different movement principles – from yoga, gymnastics, self-defence and dance to circus training, skiing and weight training. By absorbing the synergy of different elements, Joseph Pilates worked out a system that had the perfect balance of strength and flexibility to ward off dis-ease and produce fit and functional minds and bodies. Having proven the success with his own body, he then went on to help internees in a First World War camp infirmary with amazing results. He was particularly proud of the fact that none of his 'disciples' interned with him during the First World War died in the flu epidemic that claimed the lives of millions of people worldwide. He later moved to New York where he worked with dancers, sportsmen and the general public and lived very healthily without medication to the ripe old age of 87.

strength training

Strength training is the use of traditional Western exercises to increase muscular strength and improve muscle tone. Synergize™ uses the strength exercises to counterbalance the flexibility poses used in yoga.

ballet

Ballet training involves movements that use extension as a way of lengthening muscles but simultaneously strengthens muscles for a really sharp, sculpted, toned appearance. These movements are used in Synergize™ to add flow and fluidity to the movement combinations, making Synergize™ more enjoyable to perform.

the synergize™ vital ingredients

We have only to look at any dedicated Indian yogi to realize the power of yoga in improving flexibility with the tranquillity of the mind. Combine this with Chi Kung and we can achieve that inner glow from stress relief. Stir in a few tablespoons of Pilates postural realignment to prevent and ease back pain and a smidgen of ballet and strength training to increase our lean outer and inner muscle tissue (body and brain) and we have a rich cocktail designed to produce a lean and healthy, balanced mind and body equipped to handle the stresses of today.

The Synergize™ salutations and strategies outlined in this book will help lead you along the perfect journey to mental and physical synergy no matter what life throws at you. Synergize™ nourishes the mind and balances the body in a way that no other 'exercise programme' can. Say goodbye to endless repetitions or mindless movement patterns and enjoy the powerful Synergize™ principles documented in this guide especially for you to develop your own perfect and unique mind and body connection.

how is synergize™
different?

A revolutionary concept in dynamic movement, Synergize™ is an exercise programme unlike any traditional aerobics workouts in that it nourishes both the mind and body. Synergize™ inevitably initiates a discussion of functional and usable strength and flexibility as the programme relates its training methods and purposes to people's normal physical requirements for everyday activities. Often, when people work out or exercise they use an isolated training approach and have one exercise for the buttocks, another for the thighs and a separate one for the abdominals. Although a successful and proven way of exercising, this is not the only way.

body systems synergy

The human body is not a 'box of separate muscles' all working independently of each other. In fact our body systems all function in synergy with each other. The skeletal system (see page 14) provides the bone framework; the neuromuscular system provides nerve impulses and messages to initiate movement from emotions or feelings; the muscular system (see page 15) receives the messages and pulls upon the bones to provide movement; and the respiratory system extracts oxygen from the air to fuel the muscles to do their work and dispose of waste gases – a perfect working model of synergy.

functional
versus usable strength

Look at the exercise machines found in sports centres and health clubs and you will realize that they mostly work the body in straight lines. This gives us usable strength but it is not functional for everyday activities – some of our muscle groups are tight and too strong in relation to other muscle groups that are underused and weak. As you will know from vacuuming the carpet or

'The human body
is a perfect working
model of synergy'

lifting heavy items out of the boot of the car, you need to be able to access your strength in a multi-dimensional format. The body is designed to move in a complete circle, so it does not make sense to spend too long exercising in straight lines when we do not always access this type of strength for functional living.

Similarly, why perform hundreds of sit-ups as part of an exercise programme, when such an exercise clearly works only your upper abdominals (rectus abdominis) and has no synergy with other muscle groups? In everyday life you actually require the back extensors to contract with the lower abdominal muscle (transversus abdominis), to support you while lifting, running, driving, sitting at work, playing sport or even reading this book!

Synergize™ teaches you all the best exercises for functional strength, thereby maximizing your precious time.

regeneration versus degeneration of energy

The body you have today is a different breathing, living, growing organism from the one you had yesterday, will have tomorrow, next week or next year. The state of your body is influenced by a variety of factors in the same way that nature is. Just as mountains, deserts, the seasons and planets all go through cycles of regeneration and degeneration so, too, does your body. Some days you exercise, eat well and sleep lots and you feel great – you are feeding the body what it needs to regenerate bodily cells. Other days you wake up hung-over, have dull skin, are tired from too many work deadlines or you have not had the time to eat well and you feel susceptible to dis-ease – you are degenerating bodily cells.

You have the control, depending on how you live your life, to choose to regenerate or degenerate (see page 18). Synergize™ will help you become aware of both these cycles and, through the programme's movement patterns, breathing and meditations, assist regeneration of all bodily cells for the rest of your life.

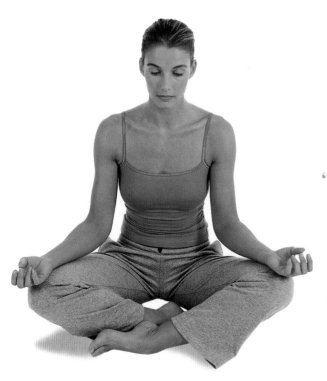

MIND STRETCH

If you have undertaken exercises or activities in the past that have made you feel even worse than when you started, it may be that the activity was simply not suited to your body or mind! Synergize™ allows you the time and space to absorb the movements and postures that feel good to you. Whatever feels natural and the easiest with effort are the exercises that will make you feel fabulous.

a new approach

Understanding and using the synergy between your brain, breath, bones and muscles is a 'global' approach to mind and body exercise that has rarely been considered before. Synergize™ will help you benefit mentally and physically from all of the programme's positive attributes for everyday *functional* use. Synergize™ recognizes that modern life is different and addresses the issues our minds and bodies really face on a daily basis. In reality this helps us to function optimally with regard to our individual environments, stresses, foods and lifestyles.

The attraction of Synergize™ lies in it being the culmination of proven Eastern and Western principles of wellbeing from over 5,000 years of research and reflective thought. It is a single realistic, successful and classical combination without any religion or deep spirituality.

'Understanding and using the synergy between your brain, breath, bones and muscles is a "global" approach to mind and body exercise.'

the skeletal system

The skeletal system makes up ten per cent of your body. It includes all the bones in your body as well as the joints that are formed as these bones attach to and move over and against each other. Synergize™ focuses on your body's core, the area from your skull to your pelvis.

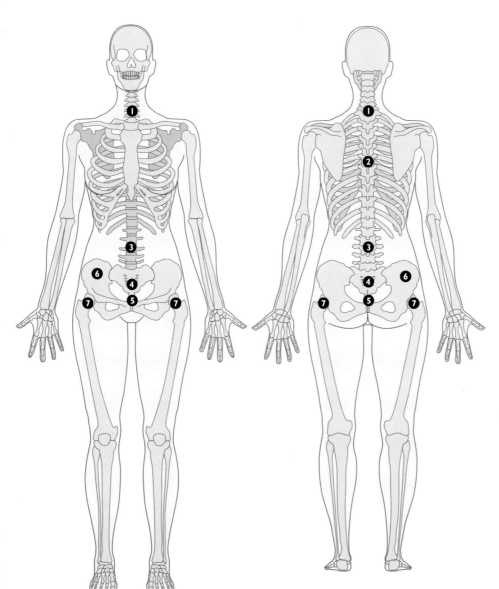

1 Cervical vertebrae – this upper section of the spine, the top seven vertebrae, is very flexible, allowing the head a wide range of movement. However, this flexibility makes the cervical spine particularly vulnerable to injury.

2 Thoracic vertebrae – these 12 vertebrae are linked to and move with the 12 pairs of ribs. The ribs form a protective cage that shields the body's internal organs from injury.

3 Lumbar vertebrae – the five vertebrae between the ribs and the pelvis bear the weight of the whole torso.

4 Sacral vertebrae – these five vertebrae eventually fuse together with the coccyx to form solid bone, at about 21 years of age.

5 Coccyx – the bottom four vertebrae of the spine. The tail.

6 Pelvis – made up of three fused bones, this solid structure supports the lower organs and connects the upper body with the lower.

7 Hip joint – ball-and-socket construction that connects the femur and pelvis.

the muscular system

Your body is made up of over 600 muscles – they provide your body with basic stability and are used to generate movement via the pull from the skeletal bones. It is important to understand how the main muscle groups work and what they do.

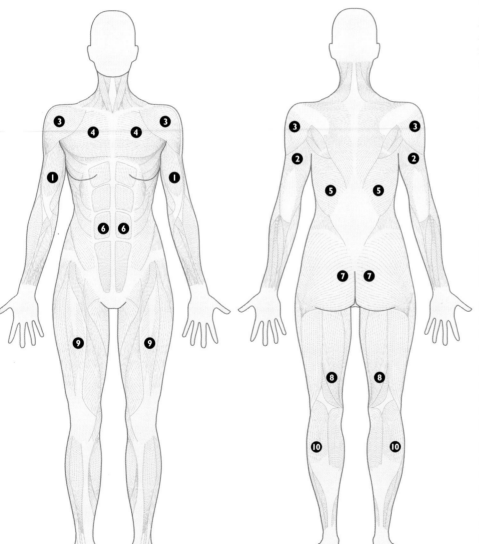

1 Biceps and **2** Triceps – muscles of upper arm. Used to move the arm.

3 Deltoid – encloses shoulder and upper arm. Used for forward and backward movement.

4 Trapezius – runs down the back of the neck and along the shoulders. Used to extend the head.

5 Latissimus dorsi – runs from the mid thoracic to the lumbar region. Helps pull the shoulders down and back and the body upwards.

6 Rectus abdominus – runs vertically down the entire front of the abdomen. This postural muscle draws the front of the pelvis upwards.

7 Gluteus maximus – forms the buttocks. Used for running, jumping and climbing.

8 Semitendinosus – runs down the middle of the back of the thigh. Used to extend the thigh and flex the leg at the knee.

9 Quadriceps – runs down the middle of the front of the thigh. It has the opposite action to the semitendinosus.

10 Gastrocnemius – forms the greater part of the calf muscles, and runs down the back of the lower leg.

the **benefits** of synergize™

The merging of the principles of traditional Eastern teachings and more modern, Western disciplines within Synergize™ offers potentially huge emotional and physical benefits. Without dieting, and without pounding your body in a hectic aerobics class, you can end up walking taller and looking a size smaller. You will be more aware of your body at work, home and play while undertaking everyday activities. Add to this your new increased confidence, calm clarity of mind and the feeling that you are in control, and you can look forward to a whole new you, inside and out.

counterbalancing physical stresses

Contemporary living imposes physical stresses upon the body that result in compensating patterns of movement that can imbalance and have negative effects on every other part of the body. For example, if you sit at a desk for eight hours a day for three years of your life and do not exercise, you will experience specific negative changes in your spine movement, hamstring flexibility, metabolism, weight, skin, scapular and muscular strength and abdominal stability.

The Synergize™ movements and breathing patterns will help you firstly to identify these stresses and secondly to counterbalance them in order for you to ooze confidence, exude elegance, look slimmer and banish backache.

feeding body and mind

Synergize™ has special positive effects on the mind, too. Besides helping counteract muscular stresses, lengthen muscle fibres and provide the body with functional strength, the Synergize™ movements and breathing exercises increase mental alertness and the ability to cope with a hectic, busy lifestyle. They work on the respiratory, circulatory and lymphatic systems – as well as the neurological, skeletal and muscular systems – ensuring a much richer supply of nourishment and elimination of toxins at cell level. It makes perfect sense that when you start to rebalance and realign the bodily systems, the core of the body will strengthen, resulting in the whole body and mind functioning more efficiently.

synergize™ benefits

The benefits to be derived from following the Synergize™ programme are wide and varied, and depend on the individual, but the following are all proven outcomes:

❖ Weight loss
❖ Improved strength and flexibility
❖ Increased lean muscle and improved muscle tone
❖ Permanent stress relief
❖ Improved concentration
❖ Better quality of sleep
❖ Enhanced awareness of body and mind
❖ Preventive measures and rehabilitation for back care
❖ Improved poise and posture
❖ Greater mental alertness and energy levels for life
❖ Better skin and hair health
❖ Stronger immunity to diseases
❖ Improved balance and coordination

safety issues

The Synergize™ programme has been researched with many experts in the UK and Australia, which is why it has proved so popular with participants whether they have back injuries, are rehabilitating an injury or are mentally and physically fit. Nevertheless, the precautions for Synergize™ are the same as for any other wellbeing, mind and body exercise programme. Check with a doctor before you embark on any exercise programme if there are any issues you are concerned about.

You will see in the Life Salutations (pages 44–109) that the flowing salutations of Dawn and Dusk require varying soothing degrees of flexion (bending) and extension work, designed to counteract the stresses of the previous movement. Less than one per cent of the population experience rapid heart rate or dizziness with these types of movements when your arms are elevated

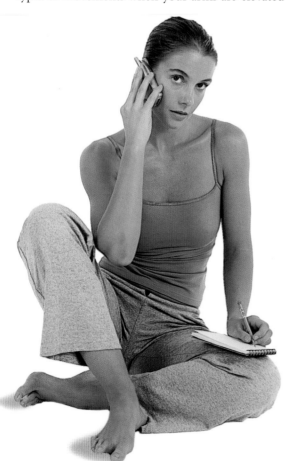

CONTRAINDICATIONS

An inverted position, including Standing Folds and Downward Dogs, should be modified to waist height only if you:
 • Are more than three months pregnant
 • Have had recent surgery
 • Suffer from any of the following conditions:
   High blood pressure
   Glaucoma
   Detached retina
   Dizziness
   Spinal injuries
   Ear problems
   Other serious illness or disease

or your head is below waist level. If you have a history of feeling uncomfortable or dizzy in these positions then you should seek medical advice *before* embarking on the exercise programme or alternatively undertake the other life exercises that can be performed in isolation.

If you have any knee injury, be careful not to hyperextend your knee and lock it straight beyond its normal limit. Always try to make sure the direction of the knee follows the direction of the foot and work on encouraging flexibility in the hips, not on forcing or straining the knees.

Some Eastern literature recommends that the inverted position should be avoided during menstruation as this is a time of contemplation to encourage *pratyahara*, a sense of withdrawal, but there are no research studies confirming this. A gentle practice of forward bends (*baddha konosana*) can sometimes ease a heavy menstrual flow.

'Synergize™ power is about taking a little time to focus on you: it is about feeling sexy and clever, sensitive and strong.'

the energy experience

The Synergize™ principles of energy preservation encompass the notion of vital inner energy, known as *chi* in traditional Chinese medicine and *prana* in Hindu teachings, to help prevent ill health and relieve current ailments. It is an important part of the Synergize™ philosophy that you understand how to 'create' as well as look after your own *chi*, to remain strong, lean, intelligent and flexible for everyday life in the 21st century. Synergize™ cultivates energy through regular practice and *experience* of the energy.

no substitute for experience

You can describe the taste of a Belgian chocolate in words – but it is only by eating one that you can experience what the term 'Belgian chocolate' actually means. In contrast to the hurried pace of the 'instant results' Western world, Synergize™ relies upon dedication and long-term consistent practice of *experience* to learn and succeed. Try stepping outside the 'quick is best' attitude and adopting a slower-but-sure approach to experiencing your results – just like the experience of the chocolate. You can look at one, you can see it is brown and soft in texture, but it is only by tasting it that you will *feel* the warm melting sensation in your mouth. This experience is your lesson and based on it you will make your own opinions and perceptions.

regeneration and renewal

Consider why it is that some winters you seem to catch every flu virus or cold doing the rounds and other years you manage to stay completely 'bug free'. This is due to the significant differences in the amount and type of cells working within your immune system at that particular time (see 'Regeneration versus degeneration of energy', page 13), which creates the difference between catching and fighting ailments. Consider, too, the state of your mind at the time and the amount of positive and negative *chi* working within, and you will understand how the mind can play a huge part in the body's responses to ill health or dis-ease.

regenerative versus degenerative lifestyles

Compare the body of a 40–50-year-old-man like Sting who adheres to a regenerative style of living and consequently looks radiant, youthful, balanced, fit, flexible and strong with that of the one-time top footballer Maradona, who drank too much alcohol and lived a degenerative lifestyle. His body became less efficient, affecting his performance on the pitch, with visible effects in his face, skin, hair and physique. His state of mind suffered negatively, too. Although he now leads more of a regenerative lifestyle, Maradona's former actions have significantly slowed down his ability to regenerate as quickly and become the player he once was.

the ancient principles of wellbeing

The ancient Eastern principles help us understand the process that allows us to stay healthy and rid the body of harmful toxins. Illness, or dis-ease, occurs when the process of body cell renewal or regeneration is disturbed through stressful modern living – for example work deadlines, poor nutrition, back pain, muscle tension, skeletal stiffness, lack of mental or physical exercise, negative habits (mental or physical) or degenerative environmental pollutants like commuting, the weather, pollution or passive smoking. The ancient healing principles regard illness as the result of a disturbed flow of *chi* around the body and the aim is to restore balance and harmony to allow the flow of *chi* – and cellular renewal – to return to normal. This method of restoring the *chi* and body cell renewal in the Western world has only ever focused on the body, not on the mind as well.

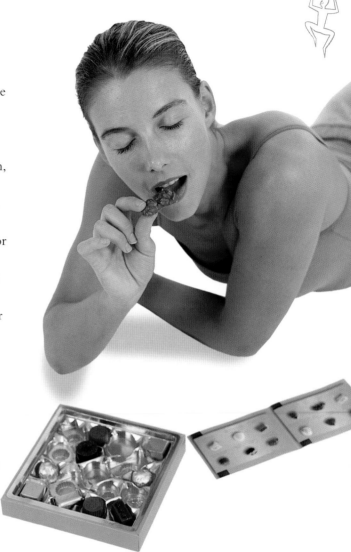

The Synergize™ programme uses breathing and meditation exercises derived from Chi Kung to *prevent* the modern-day stresses that could potentially disturb our sacred flow of *chi*, while the flexibility offered by yoga-style movements help stretch and open the body so tension is released and energy is sealed in. Synergize™ recognizes that it has been the common mistake of the Western world to treat the symptoms (mainly the body) with no concern or active thought for the cause (perceptions and anxiety of the mind). Your mind and body are hard-wired to connect, so why resist?

MIND STRETCH

The universal and global principles of *chi* as successfully used for thousands of years can be applied in an infinite number of ways. From preserving and regenerating health to achieving good fortune, they all safely sit on your own infinite and intelligent understanding that the universe is *chi*.

the importance of *chi*

The flow of *chi* is a magnificent journey that will enlighten your awareness of positive and negative *chi* and how your mind and body responds. Not all negative *chi* is referred to as 'bad' or positive *chi* as 'good'. Sometimes a balance of the two is required in order to restore the flow of *chi* and remedy the mind or body of any ills. In bereavement, for example, one experiences a sombre feeling of low ebbing energy, which allows for the flow of *chi* to facilitate the mourning process. This is not necessarily 'bad' *chi*; it is the positive process of the journey of change that has to take place in order for the *chi* to flow harmoniously through this difficult time.

meridians, *nadis* and chakras

For the sake of good health and wellbeing, the flow of *chi* must be balanced, consistent and calm. Just as a Feng Shui practitioner will research the flow of *chi* in a home and rearrange objects to remedy any blockages, energy leaks or negative *chi*, anything that negatively affects the flow of *chi* within the body or causes it to stagnate requires remedial action to restore *chi* circulation.

energy channels

Meridians are the energy channels used in traditional Chinese acupuncture and shiatsu. Akin to these are *nadis* (taken from the Sanskrit root, *nad*, meaning movement) in Hindu philosophy. They are subtle thread-like energy rivers that carry *prana* (life force) throughout the body. There are 72,000 *nadis* in the body and the key river is the *susumna*, which runs through the centre of the spine. This key river is plaited with two subsidiary *prana* rivers called Ida and Pingala.

The Ida *prana* river carries the breath of the moon (yin), which is feminine and passes through the left nostril. Its energy is maternal, nourishing, emotional and it is a calming breath. The Pingali *prana* river carries the breath of the sun (yang), which is masculine and passes through the right nostril. Its energy is vital, dynamic, rational and cleansing. These two energies relate to the balancing of the moon and the sun aspects of ourselves – in physical terms the left and right sides of the body/mind.

Through Synergize™ movement patterns and Chi Kung breathing principles all the energy rivers are regenerated and cleansed, allowing the flow of *chi* to flow through the clean rivers without blocking or limitation.

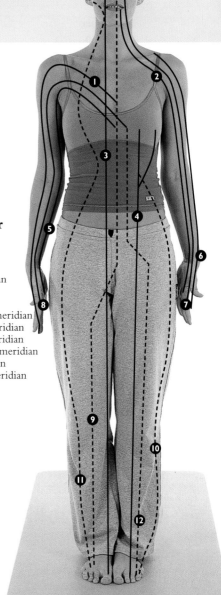

the 12 major meridians

1 lung meridian
2 colon meridian
3 stomach meridian
4 spleen meridian
5 heart meridian
6 small intestine meridian
7 triple heater meridian
8 pericardium meridian
9 urinary bladder meridian
10 kidney meridian
11 gall bladder meridian
12 liver meridian

chakras

According to Hindu philosophy, chakras are energy centres situated along the spine, linking the body with the mind. The seven chakras are placed at sacred junctions where the main *nadis* converge and plait as they weave up the *susumna* through the spine. This concept of energy is similar to the Chinese meridian system and the chakras also correspond roughly to the glands in the body's endocrine system. The latter is stimulated by hormones within the blood, which regulate the activities of our tissues and organs and play a vital role in regulating the immune system and our reaction to stress. Each of the chakras is linked to a specific gland on a physical, mental and emotional basis. If any of the chakras are out of balance through stress, inactivity or tension, this will cause a *chi* deficiency in some of the organs, which results in sluggish energy levels and can eventually lead to illness. By being aware of your chakras and energy levels you are able to detect imbalances earlier through your feelings, and avoid 'energy vampires' – stress or any ailment that saps your energy.

yin and yang

Just as we can feel the opposites of positive and negative *chi* and the important relation of each to the other, another fundamental principle of Synergize™ is the concept of yin and yang from Chinese philosophy. Although they are regarded as opposites, there is always an element of yin in yang and vice versa – hence the white dot of yang within the black dot of yin and the reverse in the yin/yang symbol.

Balancing yin (the moon, feminine, dark and passive) and yang (the sun, masculine, warm and positive) facilitates the flow of *chi* throughout our lives and the activities that we undertake. In ancient Chinese medicine areas of the body or mind processes are classed as either yin or yang and illness or stress is regarded as the result of a yin/yang imbalance. It is through our own awareness of subtle day-to-day changes in our cellular make-up and external stresses that we can track imbalances early to avoid serious illness or stress-induced burn-out.

the chakras

1 crown chakra
2 brow chakra
3 throat chakra
4 heart chakra
5 solar plexus chakra
6 sacral chakra
7 root chakra

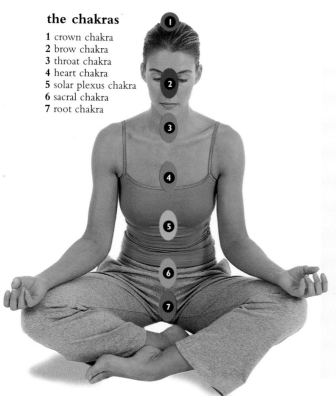

MIND STRETCH

Just as you become familiar over time with motorways and smaller roads and can drive around without a map, view your own unique awareness of your energy river system the same way. Learn how your energy feels at certain times of the day, week and year. Become aware of seasonal changes and links to your skin, hair, mood and style of dress. Learn where your energy chakras are and what they mean. This way you will know what is important for you and become a successful cultivator and driver of your own energy map and rivers.

breathing
correctly

Breathing is the very basis for life. We can go many days without food and a few without water, but without air the brain quickly becomes seriously damaged. Yet how many of us even think about our breath? We probably spend more time commuting, doing household chores, working out at the gym or worrying about work deadlines than actually consciously practising our breathing, yet there is perhaps nothing else in life that can give us so much for so little. The correct way to breathe is calmly and deeply using the diaphragm muscle and abdomen, rather than breathing shallowly from the chest or sternum as most of us do.

inner focus

Eastern-inspired philosophies have long recognized the importance of regulating the breath in order to soothe the mind and body. Deep conscious breathing strengthens the lungs, nourishes the body and steadies the mind. It creates a feeling of space within the mind for creative thoughts and reflective processes, encouraging the leading of easier, tranquil and calm successful lives. Being in a relaxed state is an important element of Synergize™ because if your breathing is shallow and rapid your mind is unable to perform as effectively, thus blocking the lesson of *experience*.

Nowadays, we are so used to 'multi-tasking' our minds to speed up our achievements we often find it impossible to think of one thing at a time. If you have been unsuccessful with meditation in the past, this may explain why you failed.

energy and conscious breathing

Energy or *chi* is called *prana* in yoga. The inhalation of breath is referred to as the cleansing wave, which increases *prana*. The exhalation is the detox wave, which eliminates impurities and makes room for more *prana* to enter the body. The aim of conscious breathing is to equalize and balance the inhalation with the exhalation, drawing the mind's focus inwards, channelling thoughts within and facilitating meditation while in motion.

We have to retrain our minds to make breathing a conscious internal effort in order to achieve balance. The positive and negative breaths will eliminate toxins and stagnant *chi*, increasing our own personal energy and *prana* through breathing alone.

In Synergize™, the mind is the driver of the *chi* energy and leads the process through visualizations and movement patterns. All Synergize™ postures are synchronized with your breath and you will learn that as we inhale we deepen the energetic charge in the body by switching on (contracting) the muscles of the trunk and core. Every single time we exhale we surrender the spine to the core, thus dissipating tension.

meditation

Although lots of spiritual schools of thought highly recommend and practise it, meditation is not a belief system. It is primarily a discipline for training your mind to a point of both deep concentration and relaxation. Think of meditation as an exercise for your mind, heart, lungs and throat, much the same as you would exercise your muscles to achieve strength or tone.

During meditation and conscious breathing, the mind becomes 'detached' from reality and enters into a state of calm and tranquil awareness in which alpha waves (the calmest of the four basic types of oscillating electrical voltages, or waves, in the brain) predominate and the body remains more alive in its natural state without imbalances from external influences or environments. This could be explained as a human *being* rather than a human *doing*, in other words recreating that calmness in the mind that feeds the body with energy from just being.

The breathing practices overleaf have been specially developed to teach you how to breathe consciously through the diaphragm and stomach. Through this type of deep diaphragmatic breathing you will be able to understand the difference between the breath you use at work or at the gym and the breath you will use for meditation and quiet time for yourself.

benefits of conscious breathing

❖ Strengthens lungs
❖ Increases energy and vitality
❖ Soothes the mind and releases stress
❖ Improves concentration
❖ Feeds the skin with nutrients and fresh energy
❖ Enhances circulation
❖ Improves fitness through efficiency of the breath
❖ Gives you a feeling of presence and actuality
❖ Improves sleep quality
❖ Soothes the thyroid, parathyroid and adrenal glands
❖ Aids digestion and removal of toxins

MIND STRETCH

A US study of 2,000 19–23-year-old students who were taught to meditate and breathe correctly found that the number of them who smoked was halved in the first six months of the trial.

The ancient yogis taught that we have been given a set number of breaths (21,600 per day) and 100 years to live. Tibetan monks claim that slow conscious breathing can result in a lifespan of 120 years.

'The breath diffuses energy through the body like waves of the sea.'

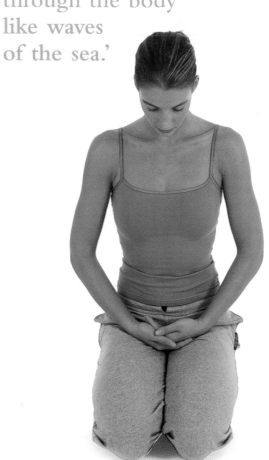

learn to
slow down

Do you feel rushed, pressurized and indecisive? You need to slow down. Try turning off the television, leaving your work behind at the end of your shift and learning the following breathing techniques. Using the diaphragm muscle and abdomen is the best way to breathe and, for the majority of the Synergize™ exercises, you need to breathe through your nose. However, conscious breathing takes practice and beginners and anyone who encounters any breathing problems should let their breath run freely without control and not try to force any unnatural changes in their breathing. Over time your practice will slow breath down anyway and you will become more comfortable.

breathing in front of a mirror

This breathing exercise will identify how you breathe and how to improve the quality of your breath by seeing yourself in the mirror.

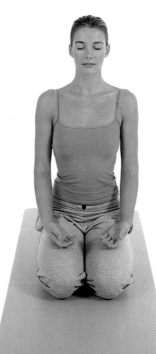

- Sit cross-legged or kneel in front of a mirror. Keep your spine long and your abdominals zipped (pulled) in to your chest. Place your hands, palms facing upwards, on the inside of your knees and relax your fingers. Breathe in through your nose and aim to fill out your chest rather than expand it upwards.

- Look at yourself in the mirror as you breathe. If you are breathing correctly you will see your chest expand and your shoulders move only slightly. If you raise your shoulders as you breathe in, this indicates that you are breathing shallowly from the chest instead of from the diaphragm, which can cause tension within the respiratory system.

- Breathing in and out through your nose, continue to take calm, full, deep diaphragmatic breaths, filling out your chest and waist. Practise for 5 minutes until you have minimized shoulder elevation when you breathe.

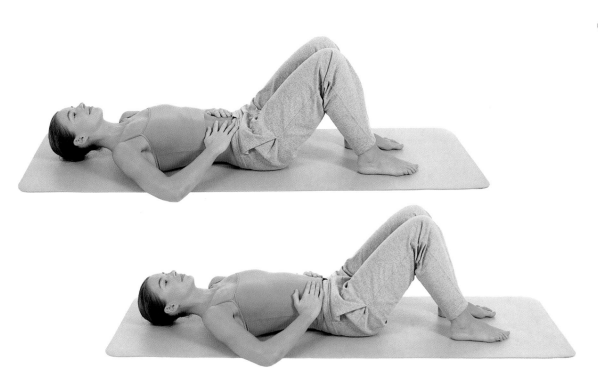

breathing while lying on the floor

Lying down (semi-supine) ensures that your back is supported by the floor and your head is centrally relaxed while you breathe deeply.

- Lie down, bend your knees so that your feet are flat on the floor and rest your hands on your abdomen. Breathe in deeply through your nose, expanding your abdomen outwards into your hands so that it rises like a loaf of bread in the oven. As you breathe out through your nose, relax and release your abdomen back to its natural position. This will encourage your abdomen to fill correctly when breathing. Practise for 5 minutes.

- When you have successfully managed to fill out your fingers with your in breath, try placing your hands slightly above your abdomen. Inhale as before and aim to expand the breath in your abdomen so that it touches your fingers. Hold on to this transition of energy for a short while. Exhale, and slowly release the abdomen back to its normal position.

- Keep practising for 5 minutes. You will sleep better in the evening and you will breathe away all the tensions and anxieties stored within the body.

water
and a healthy diet

In order for our bodies to burn fuel (the food we eat) and produce physical energy we require water as a necessary element to our existence. Another fundamental for a healthy existence is food, the quality of which makes a huge difference to our physical health, and most importantly, our brain/mind power. A diet to keep our minds and bodies healthy needs to comprise foods with a specific value for the heart and cardiovascular system, the digestive system, the brain/mind and the nervous system; organic, natural live foods that have not been contaminated by chemicals like pesticides and additives, for example.

dehydration

Our bodies require a constant balance of pure water throughout the day in order to function optimally. Without adequate water you will experience the early effects of dehydration in your throat and mouth. Body cells begin to dry up and function less efficiently, the skin dries out, causing premature ageing, and you will not be able to continue functioning at your best. These effects deplete your body of the vital energy necessary to stay well, active and radiant and you will probably encounter various subtle symptoms that often seem unrelated to simple water intake (see below).

The physical effects of dehydration are:
❖ Headaches
❖ Poor skin cell renewal
❖ Poor toxin removal
❖ Dry skin or rashes
❖ Irritability
❖ Sluggish kidneys
❖ Fatigue
❖ Bad breath

the essence of life

Water is the essence of life and by topping up the level in our bodies we replace essential mineral losses and salts.

We require six to eight glasses of pure water every single day just to stay at *base* level. Aim to have one glass in the morning and another three before lunchtime, then you won't have to feel like you are catching up for the rest of the day.

Be sensible and space your water intake out over the day and you will notice an extra subtle charge of energy throughout the day that will help you cope with life's chores much more efficiently. Remember, your body doesn't stop needing water just because the weather might be cooler.

Tea, coffee and fizzy drinks do not count as water intake as they are laden with tannins and caffeine, which strips your body of more water than it gains. So for every cup of tea, coffee or fizzy drink you need to drink two glasses of water to pay back.

eating healthily

The better balanced your diet and the less processed your food, the more efficiently your digestive system is able to work and the more effectively your blood can deliver nutrients to your entire body and brain.

By reducing your intake of wheat, dairy and meat products and following a diet more like that of our ancestors, you will be far less likely to suffer obesity- or cholesterol-related diseases. For example, concentrate on eating greens, seeds, nuts, berries, fruits, eggs, a variety of fish and seaweed if near the sea, and meat only occasionally. Similarly, eat food that is mature, in season and fresh.

Although the old-fashioned way of buying your food fresh and cooking it straight away is more time consuming than the modern supermarket culture of convenience foods, your food will be fuelling you in the best way.

good habits

Undesirable eating behaviour is usually down to habit. We often say 'yes' to a 'naughty' treat or an unhealthy item on the menu we know we like. Learn to question yourself before eating, for example: Is this food fresh and pure enough to be part of me? Am I hungry now or do I simply need a drink? In this way you can start to change your eating behaviour.

maintain a healthy weight

The simple rule of food consumption in relation to body weight is that if you eat more calories than you use up via activity, the excess calories will build up and you will put on extra weight. Many illnesses and diseases are caused by being underweight, or – as is more common in the Western world – overweight, and if you want to improve your health, you should ascertain your ideal weight and stick to it.

On a regular basis stand naked in front of a mirror. Look at yourself objectively – front and side on – and consider whether you look as fit or as healthy as you should. Decide

MIND STRETCH

Eat with intelligence and become more intelligent. A study at the Institute of Food Research in Reading in 1999 discovered that women who dieted to lose weight, didn't just lose pounds, but also lost reaction time, memory efficiency and attention span. The study found that it was not the diet itself, but the stress associated with this growing negative habit that caused a decrease in mental performance.

between the things you can change or improve and accept the things you cannot – be realistic. Take appropriate dietary action, find out where your weaknesses lie and improve them.

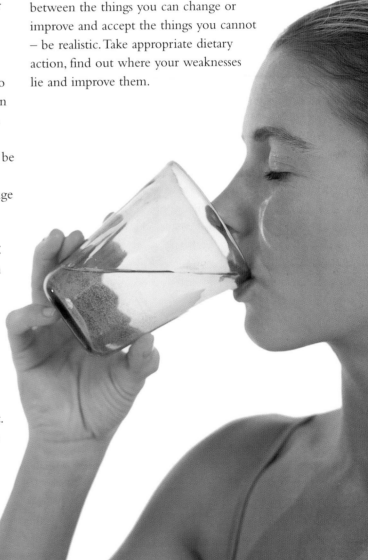

sleep and relaxation

Sleep is vital for us to remain fresh, energetic and above all alive. After oxygen and water, it is the next most important function your body needs to be able to perform, and perform well. We all feel the effects of a poor night's sleep and when we think about the causes of poor sleep we always come back to the mind and how powerful it can be in actually stopping us from dropping off to dreamland. Thinking about work, children, relationship problems, financial worries, family issues and career prospects can all play havoc with our physical ability to switch off.

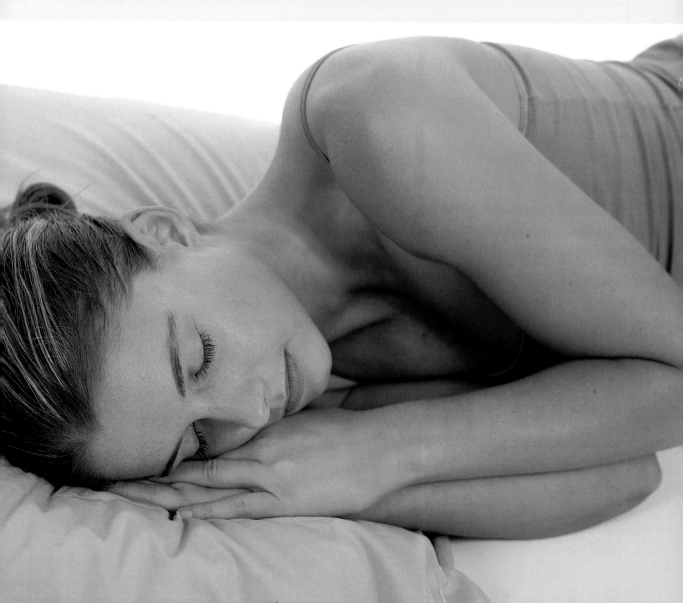

'The only devils in this world are those running around in our own heads and hearts and that is where all our battles ought to be fought.' Gandhi

rest

Sleep is one of the deepest forms of rest and is where your brain integrates the day's experiences, sorting, reflecting, filing and solving problems. Your dreams are a natural part of this process and are usually where you are at your most creative and inspirational.

Rest is a necessary function to balance active learning and the assimilation of data. Your mind needs regular breaks just as your body needs regular periods of activity. If you do not take regular mind breaks through meditation or sleep, your mind will take them anyway in the form of a loss of concentration, nervous tension and poor decision-making.

These are all ways in which your mind can insist that you take a break from whatever you are doing and balance yourself. In some extreme cases, lack of rest can lead to a nervous breakdown. In a well-exercised and well-fed body, sleep will be deep and curative, and will often provide, from an infinite source of creativity, more insights and revelations.

With Synergize™ you will learn to listen to your own body and, through the programme's meditations and breathing techniques, you will be able to make sure that the sleep you do get is of high quality.

relaxation

Many of us think we are relaxing when we enjoy an alcoholic drink or sit in front of our favourite television programme with a coffee and piece of cake, but this is sensory diversion rather than correct relaxation and many of us go to sleep with unresolved tensions.

Just as we need to process and digest food, we need to digest emotions to accept and experience them. Otherwise we accumulate mental and physical toxins, which can lead to psychosomatic mind-and-body-related disease.

The Synergize™ philosophy defines three types of tensions that create ailments and 'energy vampires':

❖ Muscular tension – affects the nervous system and causes endocrine (hormonal) imbalances
❖ Emotional tension– stemming from conflicting feelings like success/failure, happiness/unhappiness, love/hate and other suppressed, unexpressed emotions
❖ Mental tension – brought about by excessive mental activities, as in too much thinking and over-preparing

harmony

Synergize™ recognizes that balanced functioning requires harmony between the logical left side of the brain and our creative right side. This is the part that inspires artists and musicians, often leading them into a world of their own. Van Gogh, for example, painted as if he was in a dream state, Mozart composed in his sleep, while Goethe solved problems and Einstein accelerated his awareness by exploring the inner realms of the mind. Jung believed that a balanced, integrated person must be able to access the sub-conscious mind, the shadow – the part that is not seen – and bring it to light as a way of knowing oneself. The practices on pages 22–23 will help you to enjoy learning to swim into the ocean of your own sub-conscious mind via meditation or sleep.

stress and time management

Good synergy between mental and physical health relies on more than just good nutrition and exercise. It also relies upon our mind/brain and ensuring that we have the time to improve the wellbeing of both bodies and minds. How we think and feel emotionally hugely affects how we feel physically, and how fit we are physically impacts considerably on how we feel mentally. Your mental attitude has a direct correlation with both physical and mental health, and time management is a necessary requirement in the busy lives we invariably now lead.

the body's response to stress

Since the days of our earliest ancestors, our bodies have been programmed to deal with a threatening situation by going into full 'alert' mode. Hormones and energy pour into cells, preparing our bodies for immediate action – commonly known as the 'fight or flight' response. As soon as the threat has passed, the body should return to a normal state with hormone levels very quickly reverting back to base level. The problem nowadays is that we worry constantly about things, large and small – social relationships, crime, finances, health, the general state of the world, even what clothes to wear. This places a constant stress on our bodies as we are in continuous 'alert' mode, which causes physiological chaos. Eventually the immune system breaks down. This is usually the time when we might catch a cold, break out in spots or break a limb.

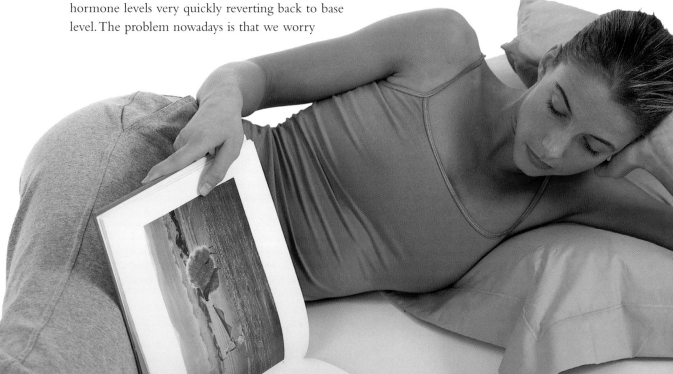

'Affording yourself just 15–30 minutes of time every day will have a bigger impact on your wellbeing than two heavy 60-minute mind and body sessions per week – try it yourself!'

managing your time

Start creating time for *you*! Your mind and body give so much back to you and for so very little in return. You deserve – and indeed *need* – your own 30 minutes of time every single day in which to do 'your thing' – something that is also conducive to inner and outer health, be it meditation, reading, exercising, cooking, stretching or window shopping. These small mental or physical 'feel good' factors will help balance your stresses.

Regard your own time as important and listen to your own needs as you would to friends, family or work demands. You are the most important, unique and amazing human being, and more powerful than any computer or machine. Maintain yourself and you will reap the rewards of boundless energy, fantastic radiant health and high productivity throughout life.

stand back from life

Imagine life as a merry-go-round, from which you can just step off and observe for a while whenever you feel the need. Try imagining for a moment that you are somebody else watching you go about your own life. Do you think that the things you are upset about are worth the worry? Whenever you start to feel stressed, standing back from life in this way will make everything seem clearer.

It is sometimes good to have a peaceful place where you can go and just think, reflect and absorb what is happening in your life right now. Some of us rush through life grasping every opportunity that knocks on our door, only to realize that if we had stopped to look at the consequences, something better or more rewarding would have revealed itself.

On the other hand, there is nothing wrong with wanting to improve your circumstances through dreams and aspirations. These are what drive you forward and keep your passions alive. The secret is to dance on the fence between living in the present moment and holding in your heart, your dreams and ambitions for the future. By standing back from life you are able to create the space in your mind to allow your dreams to progress and improve within reality.

synergize™ time

Remember that Synergize™ is all about the experience of reality and the way you want to be. Keep experimenting with different exercises and breathing patterns until you find the right strategy that works for you. You will begin to feel fitter and start having more fun – and you will then be organizing your time just right to fit in everything your mind and body require to remain balanced and healthy.

ACTIVITY PIE GAME

Draw a circle and divide it into 24 segments to represent the number of hours in the day. Colour in each segment according to the amount of time you spend doing the following:
• Sleeping
• Sitting watching television, sending emails or chatting
• Pottering about
• Brisk exercise
• Working out intensely
Look at your circle. You'll probably be very surprised to discover how much of your time is spent on your back or your bottom. Now is the time to make your time management changes.

---

bathtime
meditation

Far more than simply being the room in which you wash yourself, the bathroom is the ultimate sanctuary – a place where you can pamper yourself, blissfully cocooned away from the crazy rush of the world outside. Soaking in a hot, fragranced bath may be one of the few chances you have to indulge in private time. It stills the mind and then allows you to dream a little. How many of us discover our aspirations or make great plans while lying in the bath tub?

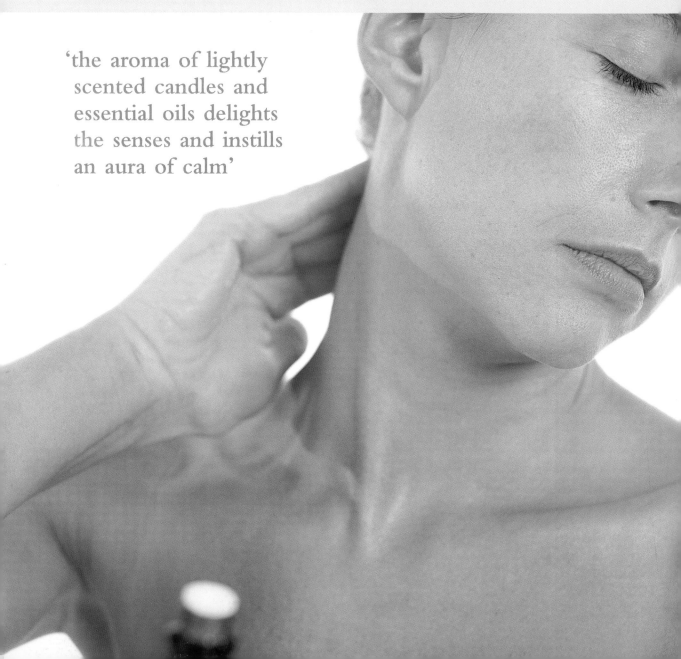

'the aroma of lightly scented candles and essential oils delights the senses and instills an aura of calm'

healing waters

Water has been called the greatest of all healers and throughout history has been used for religious purification. Today, washing is still very much associated with a renewed sense of oneself. We bathe to rinse away our stresses and tensions, and to cleanse the mind, body and spirit of negative feelings and emotions. Some experts even believe that we enjoy immersing ourselves in therapeutic baths because it returns us not only to the comfort of the womb, but also further back to our prehistoric past when we were all creatures of the sea.

essential oils

Breathing and meditation exercises are probably best done in the bath. The aroma of lightly scented candles and essential oils delights the senses and instills an aura of calm. The tiny molecules of essential oil, which are absorbed into the bloodstream directly through the skin and via capillaries in the walls of the lungs, have been scientifically proven to have specific actions on the balance of the psyche, the condition of the skin and the efficiency with which the body's internal organs function.

energizer bath breathing

✤ Light some candles and place three drops of eucalyptus essential oil in your bath.

✤ Practise inhaling smoothly for 3 seconds, hold the breath for 1 second before releasing the exhale for another 3 seconds. Close your eyes and become aware of your breathing. Count each breath and feel your abdomen rise and fall in the warm water. Visualize your organs and cells relaxing and being soothed.

✤ Allow the steam to soothe your throat; with each breath feel your body sinking into the warm water. Each breath will get slower and slower until you can begin to inhale for 4–5 seconds, pause on the exchange for a comfortable length of time then exhale for 4–5 seconds.

meditation

Not necessarily religious or spiritual, meditation is exercise for the synergy of your respiratory system (see page 23) and it clears the mind of daily clutter. The power of the mind and body connection in the sanctuary of your bathroom will recharge you and cleanse away the 'energy vampires' that sap our vital *chi* through daily activities and stress. The intrusion of thoughts is inevitable when meditating but do not try too hard. You will learn through practice to release the mind from your conscious thought via the breath. If you try to force the mind to switch off, you will actually affirm the conscious thought patterns associated with thinking this process. Recognize any recurring thoughts, let them go and draw your attention back to your breathing or the mantra you are using.

mantras

A positive mantra, or *sankalpa*, is the conscious repetition of a positive statement used to focus your life in a particular direction. It is sown like a seed in the subconscious mind where it is nurtured.

While sitting in your bath think of one single positive word or affirmation that you will achieve today, tomorrow or next week that is relevant to your goals and wishes. It could be a word such as 'peace' or a statement such as 'I will learn to relax more' or 'I will allow myself more time for me – I am important – I am strong – I can achieve so many great things this month'. Whatever it is, repeat this word or statement in your mind with determination three times. If your mind believes, you *will* achieve.

Now take five slow deep breaths in through the nose and out through the mouth, as slowly and as consciously as possible. Enjoy regenerating your body and soul. After the last breath, remind yourself of your positive word or statement and repeat it three times slowly. Fill your mind with the words. Play with the length of the words and the volume in your mind. Slowly become aware of your surroundings and open your eyes with the last word of your statement. Remain still for a few minutes and enjoy resting.

improve your
posture

Many of the problems seen by chiropractors, osteopaths and physiotherapists are related to poor posture. Posture is the very core of your bodily frame and how you carry it around day after day and year after year can significantly affect the balance of your bones and muscles. The brain remembers patterns of movement so it is the habitual way that you move, sit, walk or run that dictates the quality of your posture. By moving incorrectly you encourage problems. However, by repeating sound movement patterns and moving correctly, you can change the information that is fed to the brain. These new messages are locked into the brain's muscle memory banks and your posture can improve.

standing

A good, strong posture will help you to strengthen your muscles and lengthen your look. You will walk taller and appear more confident. The techniques used throughout the Life Salutations (see pages 44–109) will help you improve your own awareness of your standing posture. All the movements have been specially designed to counteract tension within your own body by utilizing proven and successful methods of strengthening the postural muscle groups.

negative posture

Your posture is equivalent to the chassis of a car – if the chassis is not centred the wheels will track incorrectly and the whole base of the car will be misaligned. Similarly, your pelvis, abdominals, back extensors and shoulder girdle are of paramount importance to prevent misalignment. Unfortunately many of our bodies do not function well owing to the postures that we hold and sometimes the two sides (or upper an lower segments) function differently, depending upon the habitual way we stand. When some muscles are unable to perform their functions the whole body adopts a negative posture. This makes some muscle groups compensate

for weaknesses and areas of tension. These dysfunctions are clearly reflected within our posture. By comparing the examples of good posture and bad posture we can see the significant differences. In someone displaying bad posture:

❖ The arches in the feet are collapsed
❖ An elevated hip or shoulder causes imbalances
❖ One side of the body may rotate forwards or back
❖ The pelvis and hips tilt
❖ The back rounds
❖ The chest and shoulders droop
❖ The head juts forwards or has a lean
❖ The palms face backwards or forwards

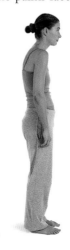
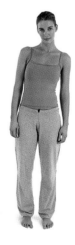

neutral alignment

Whether you are standing, sitting or lying, neutral alignment is a basic position that ensures the spine is bone-loading centrally so that pressure is applied equally to the whole spine. The neutral position is the most efficient way of engaging the lower abdominal muscle (transversus abdominis). This muscle runs horizontally from one side of the lumbar spine around to the other and is the one responsible for our true functional core strength.

Standing in neutral alignment is not the way you naturally stand and requires some practice before you really feel the benefits. You will notice over time, however, that your lower abdominals will become tighter and that you will lift and stand taller with a stronger edge. You will also have greater synergy between the abdominals, shoulder blades, feet, legs, back and head, ensuring the body stays strong and perfectly balanced for long periods of standing or sitting. This will provide you with a balanced posture, resulting in limited wear and tear on the bones and muscles for everyday activities and movements.

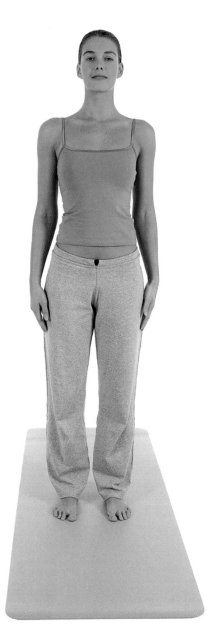

- Stand at the front of the mat with your feet together and your weight spread evenly. Your arms should be hanging loosely by your sides with your palms against your thighs. Spread your toes out on the floor like piano keys and ground the four corners of your feet. Pull your thigh muscles into the bone so that your kneecaps lift.
- Lift your upper body out of the seat of the pelvis, centring your body each side of your spine. Tuck your tailbone down and lengthen your spine upwards keeping the skin on the back of your neck wrinkle free and smooth. Feel your rib cage floating above your pelvis. Breathe deeply into your side ribs. Widen your collarbones, keeping the shoulders soft, but the armpits lifted.
- Press through the soles of your feet and lift the crown of your head towards the sky. Feel a stretch within your body – from the pelvis down, rooted into the earth, and from your pelvis upwards,

lifting your upper body towards the sky. Look straight ahead towards an imaginary horizon. Imagine putting on a belt and taking it to the end notch. You would need to breathe in and pull the lower abdominal muscle (transversus abdominis) in towards the spine. Because this would be quite uncomfortable to hold, now release your imaginary belt a few notches. The abdominals should still feel like they are zipped (pulled) in to the spine.

sitting

In the 21st century we commonly spend longer in the sitting position than we have ever done before. It is hard to believe that the chair originated as a throne for Kings and Queens as over the years it has become a necessity in our homes, offices, trains, cars and waiting rooms. We have become a nation of 'professional sitters', spending at least 10, sometimes 12, hours of our day sitting, invariably with negative postures. It is therefore no surprise that so many of us get injured doing relatively normal activities and suffer negative muscular and skeletal repercussions from all this sitting.

sitting not resting

Sitting correctly all day is static but it is demanding and certainly not a resting position. Through the Synergize™ Life Salutations (see pages 44–109) you will learn which exercises are best for you to look at your own physical demands, stresses and imbalances to prevent injuries and to perform effectively in life.

Look at and recognize the differences in posture in the two examples of sitting shown here. Through Synergize™ strength and flexibility work you will understand where your own weaknesses and tensions remain. As we spend so long nowadays sitting down it is a good idea to do it properly!

synergists and agonists

Synergists are the muscles that assist the agonists (muscle movers) to accomplish a desired action by acting as stabilizers and helping to move a specific body segment. Stabilizers hold body parts in place in a safe position so that the desired movement can occur. Synergize™ recognizes that to prevent injury and obtain optimum performance it is important to develop strength in the stabilizers simultaneously with strength in the movers.

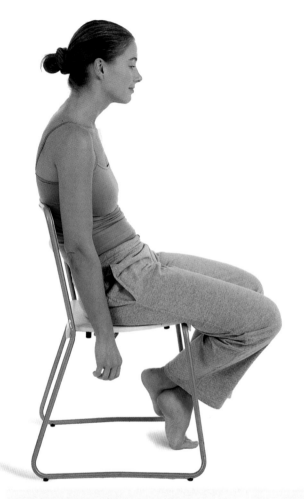

MIND STRETCH

In order to maintain a good strong posture we need to exercise the muscles needed for maintaining the correct posture. The transversus abdominal (TA), back extensors, pelvic stabilizers and muscles surrounding the shoulder girdle can all be lengthened and strengthened through Synergize™, so that maintaining a good strong posture will become easier.

JACQUELINE'S CASE STUDY

While writing this chapter I have been sitting for approximately 2 hours to maintain my creative text-writing 'trance'. My legs, particularly the backs of them, feel tight. I can feel my lower spine starting to round as I have been sitting for too long and it is getting increasingly harder to pull my transversus abdominis muscle inwards to support my spine since gravity just wants to misalign it for me. My shoulders are beginning to droop inwards from typing and again I have to pull my shoulder blades away from my ears to stop this droop from getting worse.

To add to this, my head is jutting forwards to type and because I have had my legs bent for 2 hours I feel tight, tense and uncomfortable. My body is adapting negatively to the demands of writing this book. If I did this five days a week for more than a year I probably would not be in a fit state to be asking you to read about the benefits of poor posture! However, since I am aware of these tensions and my posture I can overcome them with intelligent Synergize™ training and I can actually balance these stresses again through posture work, strength, flexibility and breathing.

good posture
for life

To reverse years of bad body use we need to go back to basics. We need to learn how to move correctly again and educate the body. With Synergize™ you do this through three stages of posture. Firstly, you will be able to bring your posture from the unconscious to your conscious mind. Secondly, with practice, you will be able to feel taller and walk longer. Lastly, it will become habit and this should be your goal – your desired outcome. Your nervous system will take these new habit messages on board and reorganize itself as a result of your improved movement.

posture exercises

Try the postural exercises here (see pages 39–43) to begin raising your own awareness. It is when these activities are repeated with awareness and intent that they are no longer a habit. With this insight, tasks can be mastered with clarity and success.

The exercises will teach you how to raise your own awareness of the deep stabilizing muscles of your pelvis and spine – the transversus abdominis, pelvic floor and multifidus muscles. In order to achieve the best possible stability of the trunk through daily activities you will also learn to master engaging these important muscle groups together in synergy with one another. These exercises will not take you long, but if you perform them daily you will notice an amazing new sense of tone and tension in the lower abdominal area and you will become much stronger and less prone to injury or back pain. Practise in front of a mirror as much as possible to see, as well as feel, the movements.

synergize™ stages of posture

There are three Synergize™ stages to the process of re-educating the body to move correctly:

♣ Awareness – thinking about good movement
♣ Practice – practising good movement
♣ Muscle memory – the new movements will become automatic and habitual

Take time to practise and you will experience these three stages of posture.

pelvic elevators

This simple yet effective exercise will teach you how to control engaging your pelvic floor to 30 per cent. This will help you to sustain a good neutral alignment in your core.

watch points

When you pull up to your second floor you should feel the deep lower abdominal muscle engage. This is your transversus abdominis muscle switching on (contracting). Your transversus is responsible for true abdominal strength and will facilitate your core by providing you with a girdle of strength.

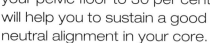

- Stand squarely with your weight evenly over your feet. Imagine that your pelvic floor is like an elevator in a building. Breathe into your lungs and lengthen through the spine. As you breathe out, draw up the muscles of the pelvic floor as if you were trying to prevent the flow of urine and take your imaginary pelvic elevator to the first floor of the building (10 per cent). Breathe in and release the elevator back to the ground. Repeat lifting to the second (20 per cent) and third floors (30 per cent), ensuring you release and come back to normal in between.
- Keep this action low and gentle, aiming to pull in around 30 per cent – pull in too much and your anal sphincter muscles will contract too tightly, causing discomfort.
- Complete 3 times, pausing at each floor for 3–5 breaths.

prone pull-in

The prone pull-in exercise will improve your posture by using the floor as a measure of your ability to pull the abdominals into the spine.

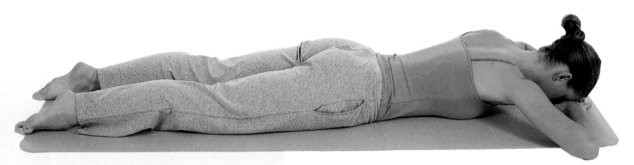

watch points

There should be no movement in your spine. Activate your movement through the internal dynamics of the pulling-in sensation of your abdominals. This synergy of abdominals will help to create a relationship with the spine during more complicated or more difficult positions.

- Lie on the floor face down. Rest your head on your folded hands, relaxing your shoulders. Move your legs to shoulder width apart. Breathe in to prepare your body for the exhalation, breathe out and zip (pull) in and hollow your lower abdominals off the floor. Imagine a drawing pin or a piece of holly beneath your belly button that you do not want to touch. Do not tighten your buttocks. Breathe in and release.
- Repeat 5–10 times, holding for the length of a breath each time.

kneeling zip-ups

Once you have managed to find your neutral alignment via the 30 per cent pelvic floor method, practise zipping your transversus abdomen into your spine to strengthen your abdominal control in varying positions.

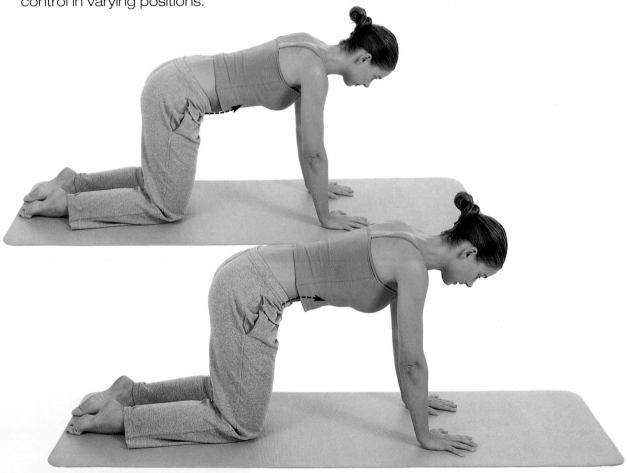

watch points

Keep the spine stabilized and do not allow it to move. If the spine moves this is an indication that you have moved out of your neutral alignment.

- Kneel on all fours with your hands directly beneath your shoulders and your knees directly in line with your hips. Keeping your shoulders drawn in, lengthen your head away from your tailbone. Your pelvis and spine should be in neutral alignment.
- Breathe in to prepare your body for the exhalation then breathe out and pull your abdominals towards the spine. Your back should not move at all. Breathe in and release.
- Repeat 5–10 times.

plumblining

This is a simple, yet effective, exercise to ensure that you are standing correctly.

watch points

Watch for rounding of the shoulders or middle back. Ensure that your 'B' line (bikini/belt line) is engaged and pulls the transversus abdominis muscle inwards to support your core. Be aware of any natural hinging forwards through the hips.

- Stand straight and ground the four corners of your feet, imagining there are tree roots attached to your heels and toes that go deep into the ground. Visualize a drawing pin underneath the arches of your feet and contract your thighs and buttocks to lift the fleshy thigh muscles out of the knees.
- Now imagine there is a tail attached to your tailbone, which is very heavy and long. It pulls down on the end of your spine and counteracts any leaning forward that you may have done while standing in the past.
- Imagine a piece of string attached to the crown of your head. It extends upwards to the sky, stretching your spine a little longer and making you feel taller and longer. This is the 'plumbline', which travels down through the spine to the pelvis.

stability slides

This posture will teach you how to stabilize the pelvis in neutral while the limbs are moved for everyday activity. You have mastered the breathing, the correct alignment of the pelvis, spine and centre and stabilizing and now you will learn how to add movement and how to coordinate the synergy of everything together. It is just like learning to drive a car and will soon become automatic within your own muscle memory of the mind. The learning journey of this process is a fantastic way to bond the mind and the body as it stimulates the communication between the physical and mental processes – mind and body exercises.

watch points

If you cannot breathe in and maintain a strong core, then take an extra breath and return your leg on the out breath. Your breath is your pacer. The slower and more consciously you breathe, the better the mind and body connection.

- Lie on your back with your pelvis in neutral and your tailbone lengthened. Place your hands on your pubic bone and hip bones in a triangle and make sure they are level.
- Inhale and prepare. Exhale, zip in your abdominals to hollow the belly and simultaneously slide one leg along the floor away from you. Keep the lower abdominals engaged and your pelvis level and stable. Imagine that throughout these moves you have balanced on your pelvis a bowl of water which you must not spill on yourself. Breathe into your lower ribs and return your leg to the start position, keeping your stomach scooped out and hollow.
- Repeat slowly 5 times on each leg.

life salutations

dawn
salutation (see pages 46–55)

The Dawn Salutation prepares the mind and body for the day ahead by harnessing energy stores and ridding the mind and body of 'negative' *chi*. It is a fluid combination of movement patterns, which performed for as little as 15 minutes have been proven to recharge energy levels and strengthen your mind and muscles ready for optimum performance for the day ahead. The breath is an important aspect of the Dawn Salutation in awakening the mind, body and soul to help achieve total harmony between them. Breathing should be slow and conscious with minimal tension and force, to thread the movements of the salutation together.

❖ The Dawn Salutation will produce most benefits when performed between 5 and 12 times in the morning before breakfast every day.
❖ This should take you no longer than 5–15 minutes.
❖ Try to ensure as much natural light as possible in your space to stimulate the feeling of energy and positivity.
❖ Ensure you have prepared room in which to work and have adequate padding for the floor positions prior to starting.

strength
salutation (see pages 56–73)

In Synergize™, movement is initiated from the inside, meaning that we move from the pelvis and the spine – the central core of the body – rather than from outer muscle strength. Synergize™ strength postures stretch, lengthen and tone muscles rather than contracting and tightening them. Use your breath consciously with the step-by step instructions given and repeat the movements until they become more natural through practice. The strength salutation begins with a *prana* flow routine that will raise your body temperature while increasing the amount of energy flowing into the body in preparation for the strength exercises that follow.

❖ The exercises can be done according to muscle preference but you are advised to perform between two and five sets of 8–12 repetitions, at least twice a week.
❖ Some of the exercises offer three levels for you to work through – level 1 being the easiest and level 4 the more advanced option.
❖ Take your time with these moves and if they feel unnatural you are probably working at an incorrect level.

The Life Salutations in this chapter will help you learn various combinations of movements for counteracting the stresses encountered on a daily basis.

stress-free
salutation (see pages 74–89)

This series of exercises aims to improve the way in which you deal with stress-related symptoms. The reasons for stress are many and varied and can include conflict at home or work, poor working or living conditions, high work load, relationship problems, feelings of being undervalued, lack of personal responsibility or seemingly trivial daily hassles. Take small steps to offload the stress in your life so as to take control. You do not need to do the entire sequence of stress-free exercises every time – you can start with just two or three. It is better to take your time learning the exercises properly and finding your own natural energy with them rather than rushing and trying to learn them all.

✤ Make the exercises your own and perform them every day to clear any blocked pressure or energy within you.
✤ You will notice how much fresher and in control you feel after performing these exercises regularly over a period of time.
✤ Your skin will begin to glow. You will look younger and your body will feel lighter and longer and free of the heavy tension that can sometimes deplete your energy stores.

dusk
salutation (see pages 90–109)

The Dusk Salutation is best done in the evening as it will help you switch off from your day. It will also help to improve flexibility, your muscle tone and condition, and will assist restful sleep. The physical movements are guided by your breathing. If you practise the breathing cues to go with each movement of the Dusk Salutation you will achieve peace of mind at the same time. Practise letting go of your breath and you will find that your body will follow fluidly.

✤ Perform the salutation 5–10 times in the evening and affirm in your mind the good things that have happened in your day as you breathe in.
✤ Fill your body with energy and allow it to stretch and free any tension.
✤ Practise each section of the Dusk on its own so that you can then learn the whole salutation correctly.

dawn salutation

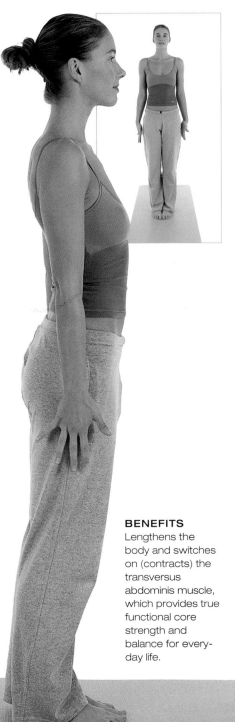

BENEFITS
Lengthens the body and switches on (contracts) the transversus abdominis muscle, which provides true functional core strength and balance for every-day life.

1 neutral alignment

- Stand at the front of the mat with your feet together and your weight spread evenly. Your arms should be extended by your sides with your palms against your thighs. Spread your toes out on the floor like piano keys and ground the four corners of your feet. Pull your thigh muscles into the bone so that your kneecaps lift.

- Lift your upper body out of the seat of the pelvis, centring your body each side of your spine. Tuck your tailbone down and lengthen your spine upwards keeping the skin on the back of the neck wrinkle free and smooth. Feel your rib cage floating above your pelvis. Breathe deeply into your side ribs. Widen your collarbones, keeping the shoulders soft, but the armpits lifted.

- Press through the soles of your feet and lift the crown of your head towards the sky. Feel a stretch within your body – from the pelvis down, rooted into the earth, and from your pelvis upwards, lifting your upper body towards the sky. Look straight ahead as if towards an imaginary horizon.

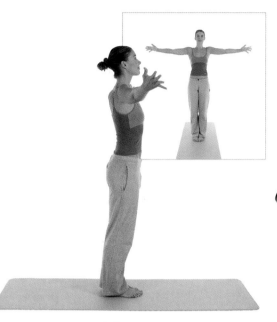

2 transition

- Inhale freely and fill your lungs, while raising your arms, palms up, out to the sides, and bending your knees slightly as you continue to raise your arms above your head, keeping them straight.

BENEFITS
Fills the body with energy and releases tension in the body through the extension of the pose.

3 mountain pose

- Still inhaling, take your arms above your head, keeping them long and strong to maintain the flow of energy. Keep your head in a central position.

4 transition

- Exhale, and begin to hinge forwards from the hips, taking the arms out to the sides. Imagine diving off a cliff.

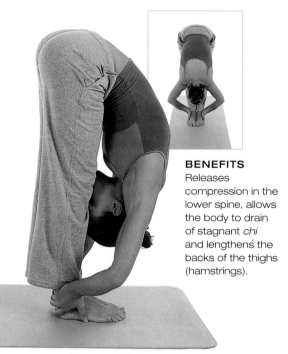

BENEFITS
Releases compression in the lower spine, allows the body to drain of stagnant *chi* and lengthens the backs of the thighs (hamstrings).

BENEFITS
Good for functional core stability as the abdominals and back extensors are worked together.

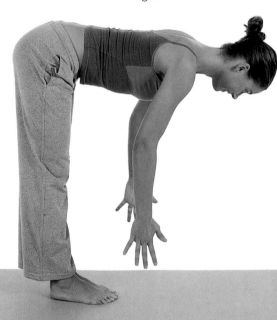

5 standing fold

- Continue to slowly exhale, pulling your belly in towards your spine, as you begin to fold the body into two as if letting air out of a lilo, your arms hanging below your head.
- Imagine that you are diving into water and push your arms behind you in a circular motion as though to swim back up to the water's surface after your dive. Allow your back to round in the last third of the movement to release any compression in the discs and lower spine.

6 active back extension

- Inhale through your nose and contract your abdominals as you begin to raise your shoulders to hip height.
- Keep your neck in line with the rest of the spine, looking straight down. Keep the whole of your feet pressed into the floor and contract the front of your thighs (quadriceps) to initiate a good stretch in the backs of the thighs (hamstrings).
- Ensure your back is flat by pulling your shoulder blades away from your ears. This position is great for core stability and strengthening your shoulders for good posture. If you find this difficult you can support your core by placing your hands on your thighs for assistance.

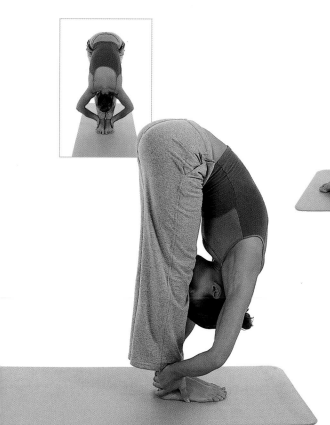

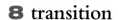

8 transition

- Inhale and place your hands on the floor by bending your knees.
- Exhale and kneel first on your right leg then on your left leg so that you are kneeling on all fours.

7 standing fold

- Slowly exhale through your mouth and extend your arms forwards to lead your body back down to the standing fold posture.
- Keep your shoulders away from your ears – imagine your shoulders are on fire and you do not want to burn your ears. Release your spine.

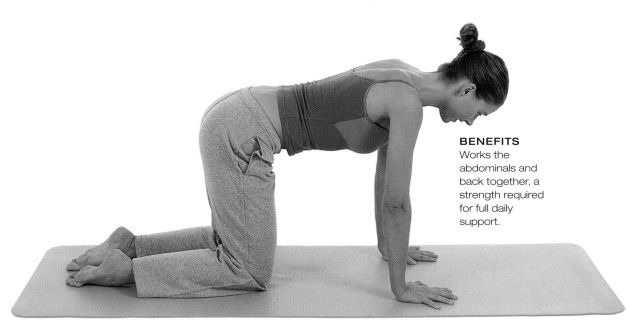

BENEFITS
Works the abdominals and back together, a strength required for full daily support.

9 table-top active

- Pull your belly in towards your spine or engage your pelvic floor 30 per cent, ensuring that you still have a slight natural curve in the base of your spine.
- Engage the shoulder girdle by lifting and pulling your shoulders away from your ears, releasing any neck tension – imagine you are trying to hold a piece of paper between your shoulder blades (scapulas). Your chest will open and lift as a result.
- Ensure your palms are flat on the floor and your knees in line with your hips. Breathe comfortably while maintaining a neutral spine.

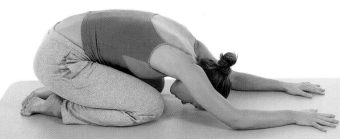

10 transition

- Inhale gently, filling your lungs like two balloons. As you exhale, start to ease your buttocks down towards your heels.
- While exhaling, release your buttocks as low to your heels as possible. Lean forwards until your head touches the ground, stretching your arms out along the ground in front of you. This posture will stretch the muscles of the spine as well as relaxing the body.

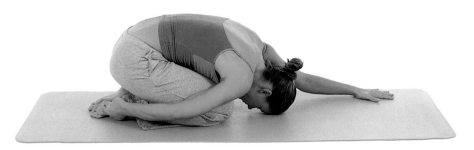

11 transition

• Release one arm behind you and relax the back of the hand on the ground, the palm facing upwards to absorb energy. Allow the fingers to relax and cup. This lets the shoulder to relax and frees it from the elevation and tension experienced at stressful times.

BENEFITS
Releases pressure in the lower spine and allows the body to rest.

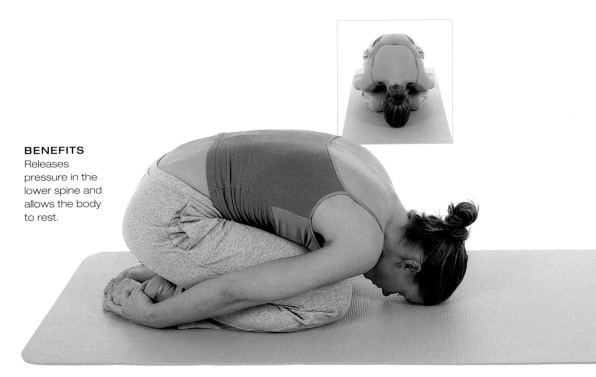

12 child pose

• Resting more heavily on your heels, tuck both your arms away behind you, with your palms facing upwards.

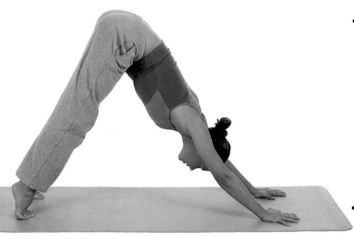

13 transition

- Inhale and take your weight on to your arms. Keep your shoulders away from your ears to strengthen the scapular and shoulder girdle postural muscles. The scapular muscles (scapulae), which are attached to the shoulder blades, pull the bones of the shoulder girdle into position and are responsible for keeping your posture tall and balanced. If your scapular muscles are weak then your shoulder girdle collapses forward resulting in poor posture.
- Lift your tailbone to the sky, pulling the 'B' line (bikini/belt line) inwards. Contract your thighs and lift your kneecaps. Lift your heels off the floor, lifting up through the arches of your feet and lengthening your ankles. Extend through your hips, freeing your pelvis of any forward flexion.
- Take your weight through your fingers as well as the heels of your hands.

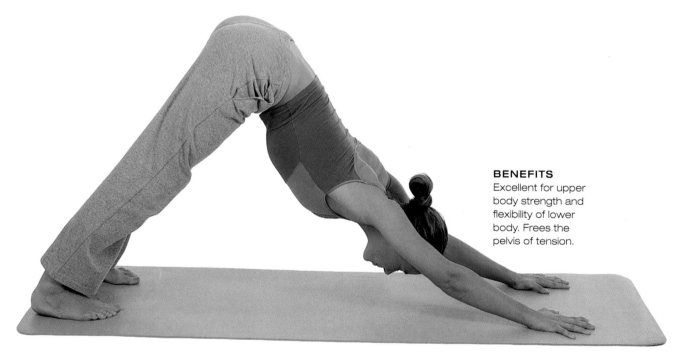

BENEFITS
Excellent for upper body strength and flexibility of lower body. Frees the pelvis of tension.

14 downward dog

- Exhale, and ease your heels back to the floor.
- Use your breath to dissipate any tension with the movement. Hold for 3–5 breaths.

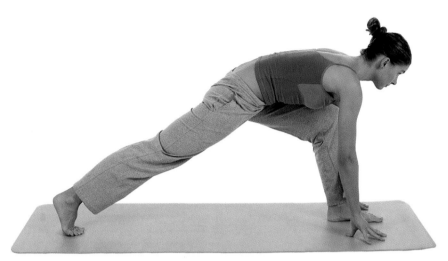

15 transition 1

- Inhale and step forwards, placing your left leg between your hands. Keep your chest lifted and look forwards and down.

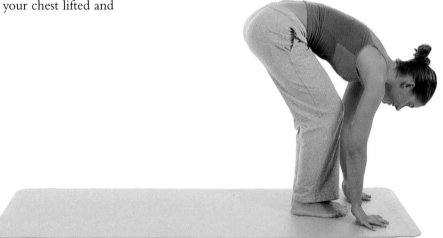

16 transition 2

- Finish off the inhale and step the right leg forwards so that your feet are between your hands, hip distance from each other.
- Keep your knees bent for support and hollow out your belly to support your spine.

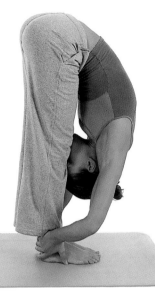

BENEFITS
Releases compression in the lower spine, allows the body to drain of stagnant *chi* and lengthens the backs of the thighs (hamstrings).

17 standing fold

- Exhale and relax the spine in a folded position. If you wish to progress the standing fold stretch you can either place your hands on the floor or ease the chest further by grasping gently behind the back of your ankles.
- Relax your head and exhale any tension you may be experiencing.

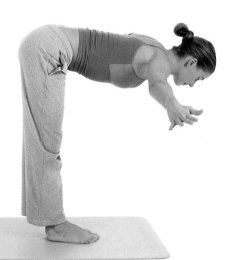

18 transition

- Inhale and hollow out your belly, raising your arms out to the side. Bend your knees slightly on your way up to support your spine.

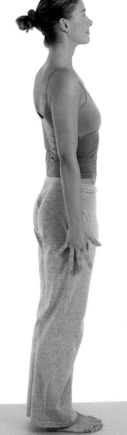

19 mountain pose

- Continue to inhale slowly until your arms are straight up above your shoulders. Keep your fingers long and strong and relax the tension in your shoulder blades (scapulas) by lifting and pulling your shoulders away from your ears.
- Maintain neutral alignment, as per Step 1, and keep your tailbone tucked underneath the pelvis with your abdominals pulled inwards.

BENEFITS
Fills the body with energy and releases tension in the body through the extension of the pose.

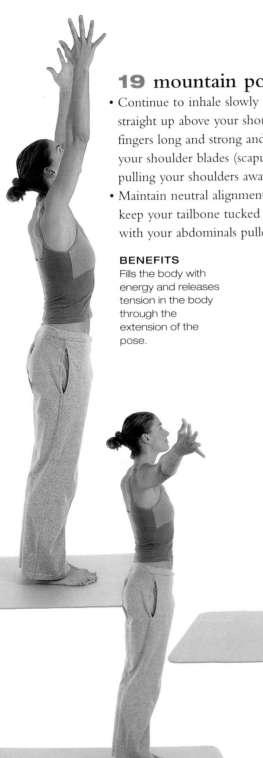

BENEFITS
Lengthens the body and switches on (contracts) the transversus abdominis muscle, which provides true functional core strength and balance for everyday life.

21 neutral alignment

- Exhale and release your arms down to your sides, your palms against your thighs and your neck relaxed in the centre of your shoulder girdle.
- Imagine putting on a belt and breathing in so as to accommodate the innermost notch. Then release your imaginary belt a few notches so that the waist is kept small and the abdominals engaged but the position is comfortable enough to hold with effort.

20 transition

- Exhale and release your arms back down out to the sides.

strength salutation
prana flow routine

This ancient sequence of simple movements is called a half vinyasa in yoga. It is designed to increase the amount of energy flowing through the body in preparatioin for the toning effects of the strength salutation. Perform the exercise 5–8 times.

BENEFITS
Opens the joints, strengthens the muscles, increases the body's temperature and melts fat deposits.

1 neutral alignment

- Stand at the front of the mat with your feet together and your weight spread evenly. Your arms should be hanging loosely by your sides with your palms against your thighs. Spread your toes out on the floor like piano keys and ground the four corners of your feet. Pull your thigh muscles into the bone so that your kneecaps lift.
- Lift your upper body out of the seat of the pelvis, centring your body each side of your spine. Tuck your tailbone down and lengthen your spine upwards making sure that you keep the skin on the back of your neck wrinkle-free and smooth. Feel your rib cage floating above your pelvis. Breathe deeply into your side ribs. Widen your collarbones, keeping the shoulders soft, but the armpits lifted.
- Press through the soles of your feet and lift the crown of your head towards the sky. Feel a stretch within your body – from the pelvis down, rooted into the earth, and from your pelvis upwards, lifting your upper body towards the sky. Look straight ahead as if towards an imaginary horizon. Engage pelvic floor 30 per cent, or pull navel to spine.

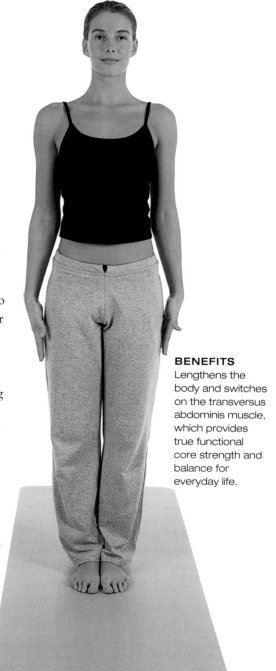

BENEFITS
Lengthens the body and switches on the transversus abdominis muscle, which provides true functional core strength and balance for everyday life.

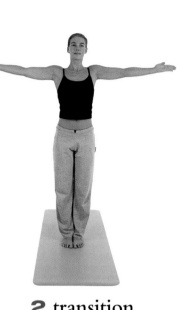

2 transition
- Begin to inhale calmly through your nose and lift your arms up and out to the sides. Hold on to your core connection and keep your pelvis tucked slightly.

BENEFITS
Releases compression in the lower spine caused by long bouts of sitting or standing and improves blood flow to the upper body. Lengthens the backs of the thighs (hamstrings).

3 mountain pose
- Lengthen your arms and take them straight above your head. Keep your fingers long and strong to recharge energy. Your hands should be level with your shoulders and your feet grounded into the earth.

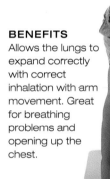

BENEFITS
Allows the lungs to expand correctly with correct inhalation with arm movement. Great for breathing problems and opening up the chest.

4 standing fold
- Exhale, and begin to hinge forwards from the hips, taking the arms out to the sides. Imagine diving off a cliff.
- Continue to exhale through the mouth, pulling your belly in towards your spine, and folding your body in half while hinging from the hips. Use the abdominals to support your spine.

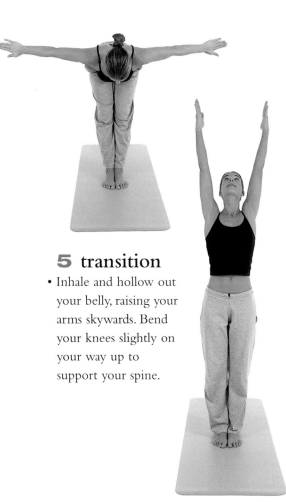

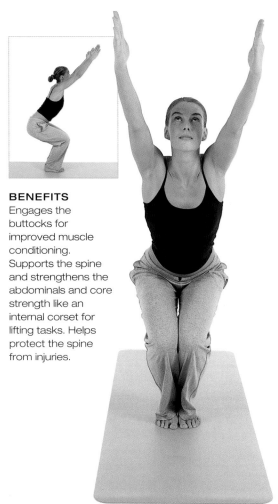

BENEFITS
Engages the buttocks for improved muscle conditioning. Supports the spine and strengthens the abdominals and core strength like an internal corset for lifting tasks. Helps protect the spine from injuries.

5 transition

- Inhale and hollow out your belly, raising your arms skywards. Bend your knees slightly on your way up to support your spine.

6 transition

- Inhale and, bending your knees slightly, push up through your legs and buttocks to a standing posture.
- Pull your belly in towards your spine and ensure your arms are long and strong. Drive (press) your legs into the floor and extend upwards through your torso.

7 chair

- Keeping your legs strong, exhale and lower your buttocks into the Chair position. (Imagine sitting on a chair but pressing your buttocks back. Keep your knees together and stretch your arms up in line with your body, pulling your shoulder blades away from your ears to broaden your collarbones and open your chest.) Hold the position for 3–5 breaths to get you really warm.
- Drive through (press down) the four corners of your feet keeping your buttocks switched on (contracted) and lifted. Lift your rib cage away from your pelvis and pull your belly in towards your spine.
- Bring your hands out to the sides to make the arms feel lighter and easier to hold, and pull your shoulder blades away from your ears.
- Keep the arches of your feet lifted and feel your breath while being aware of your body dynamics. Hold the position for 3–5 breaths.

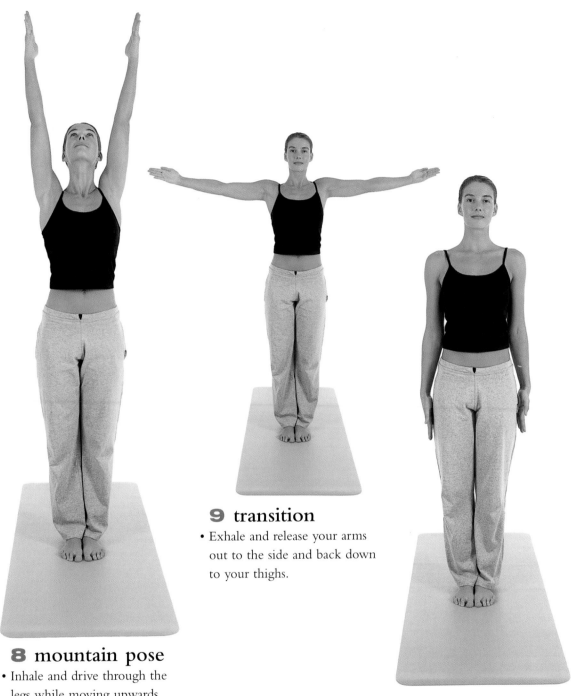

9 transition
• Exhale and release your arms
out to the side and back down
to your thighs.

8 mountain pose
• Inhale and drive through the
legs while moving upwards.
• Keep your fingers long, strong
and soft. Your thighs should
be switched on and your
kneecaps high.

10 neutral alignment
• Continue to exhale, making sure
that your chest remains lifted, and
return your arms to your sides.
Your feet should still be together
and your pelvic floor should still
be engaged by 30 per cent.

ballet lunge

Repeat the ballet lunge 8–10 times on each leg. Rest in between stretching each leg.

BENEFITS
Strengthens buttocks, abdominals and back extensors through stability and balance work. You will also experience an improvement in muscle tone and condition of the thigh muscles through hip extension and muscular work.

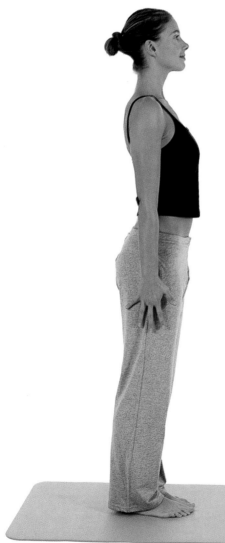

1 neutral alignment

- Stand at the back of the mat with your feet together and your weight spread evenly. Your arms should hang loosely by your sides with your palms against your thighs. Spread your toes out on the floor like piano keys and ground the four corners of your feet. Pull your thigh muscles into the bone so that your kneecaps lift. Engage your pelvic floor 30 per cent or pull in your traversus abdominals.
- Lift your upper body out of the seat of the pelvis, centring your body each side of your spine. Tuck your tailbone down and lengthen your spine upwards keeping the skin on the back of your neck wrinkle-free and smooth. Feel your rib cage floating above your pelvis. Breathe deeply into your side ribs. Widen your collarbones, keeping the shoulders soft, but the armpits lifted.
- Press through the soles of your feet and lift the crown of your head towards the sky. Feel a stretch within your body – from the pelvis down, rooted into the earth, and from your pelvis upwards, lifting your upper body towards the sky. Look straight ahead as if towards an imaginary horizon. Engage pelvic floor 30 per cent or pull navel into the spine.

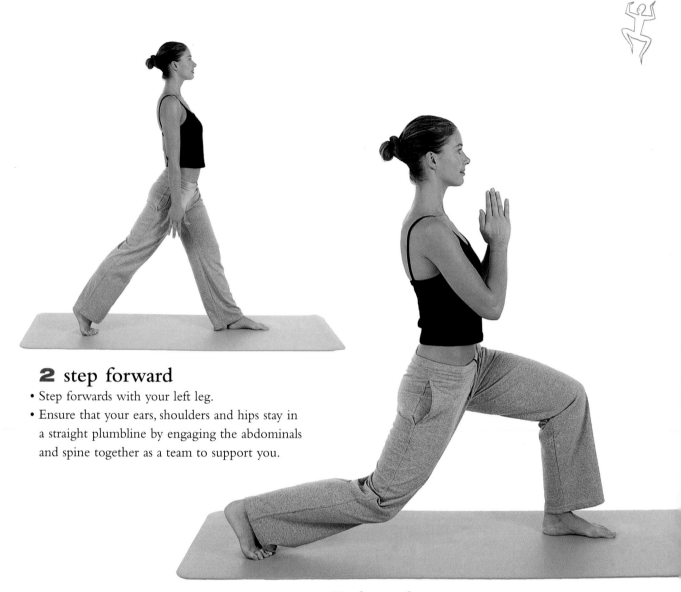

2 step forward
- Step forwards with your left leg.
- Ensure that your ears, shoulders and hips stay in a straight plumbline by engaging the abdominals and spine together as a team to support you.

3 drop down
- Both feet should be facing forwards. Hold your hands in prayer pose – together in front of your chest, a position used by the ancient yogis to focus concentration and centre the mind and body.
- Inhale and lunge downwards with your right knee towards the floor as far as is comfortable, ensuring that your knee does not touch the floor.
- Switch on the buttock muscles (gluteals) in both legs. Keep your torso extended upwards and look forwards. There should be enough room for an apple or orange to rest behind the back knee. Imagine you are moving downwards like an elevator not forwards like an escalator.

Levels of difficulty

Step 4 offers three levels for you to choose from. Use the level that feels natural to you. You will naturally gravitate to more advanced positions as you adjust to the patterns of movement.

4 level 1 (just starting out)

• As you exhale, drag through your back foot and drive up through the front foot. Come into a balancing position on your big toe, keeping the rest of your body in a long full-body leaning position. Do not tilt from the hips. A full body lean is sufficient to avoid back hyperextension.

4 level 2 (getting stronger)

• As you exhale, pull your belly in towards your spine and press through your front foot into a leg balance with the back foot slightly off the floor. Keep looking forward at the horizon.

'a slow exhale will give you
time to focus your mind'

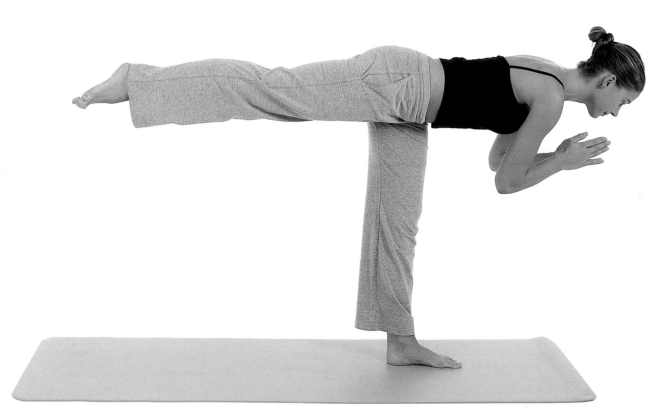

4 level 3 (strong)

- As you exhale, press through the front foot and
  contract the thigh muscle in the supporting leg. A
  slow exhale will give you time to focus your mind
  into your core and buttocks to balance.
- Press forwards into the Stork pose, whereby both
  your head and your back foot are in line with your
  hips, as you balance on a completely straight leg.
  Hold for 3–5 breaths for extra buttock toning.

V-sit stabilizer

Perform the exercise 8–12 times for a minimum of two sets at your chosen level. Hold the positions for 3–5 breaths. There are four levels for you to choose from. Use the level that feels comfortable to you. You will naturally gravitate to more advanced positions as you adjust to the patterns of movement.

BENEFITS
Strengthens the abdominals and improves synergy between upper and lower muscle and bone groups.

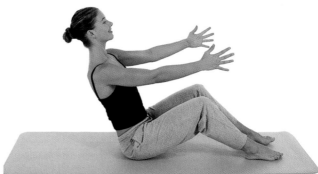

level 2 (getting stronger)

• Inhale and prepare. While exhaling release both hands one at a time so that they are level with your shoulders. You now have the extra weight of your arms to hold without letting your abdominals 'dome'. Hold for 3–5 breaths and relax.

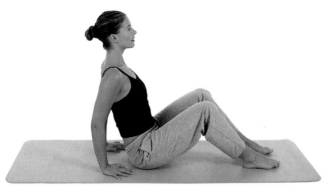

level 1 (just starting out)

• Adopt the V-sit position whereby you sit with your spine in neutral and your knees bent, with your feet a comfortable distance from your bottom. Your neutral spine forms one edge of the 'V' and your thighs the other. Place your hands behind you, palms facing inwards or outwards – whichever is the most comfortable for you.

• Draw your shoulder blades down the spine towards your pelvis and lift and open your chest. Keep your head neutral on the horizon.

• Pull your belly in towards your spine and flatten out your abdominals to ensure they do not 'dome' (bulge out). Breathe comfortably and hold for 3–5 breaths.

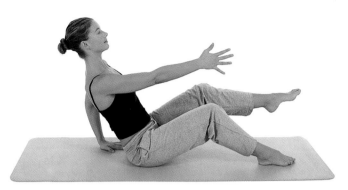

level 3 (strong)

- Inhale and prepare. Exhale and lift your right arm in front of you.
- Inhale and exhale again to lift your left leg off the floor using your hip as a hinge. Keep your feet long and your chest open. Keep pulling your abdominals inwards like an internal corset.
- Hold for 3–5 breath. Repeat on both sides.

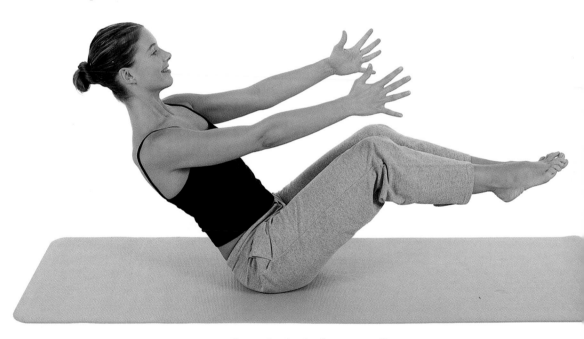

level 4 (advanced)

- Inhale and prepare. Exhale and lift both arms out in front of you. Inhale and prepare. As you exhale, lift your right leg then left leg off the floor also.
- Tilt back slightly through the sit bones (the two buttock bones beneath the fleshy muscle and fat of your bottom) and ensure that your back stays long and strong like a surfboard. Breathe slowly for 3–5 breaths then release and relax.

side plank

Perform the exercise 8–12 times for a minimum of two sets on each side at your chosen level. Hold for 3–5 breaths. There are three levels for you to choose from (level 3 has two steps). Use the level that feels comfortable to you. You will naturally gravitate to more advanced positions as you adjust to the patterns of movement.

BENEFITS

Tones and strengthens the sides of your waist, back extensors and core for lifting to the sides and for lateral strength.

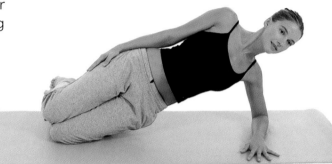

level 2 (getting stronger)

- Lie on your left side on the floor, inhale and prepare.
- Exhale and lift your left hip off the floor as before. Place the weight of your right arm on the outer thigh of your right leg.
- Keep your head in line with your spine and pull your waist in tightly. Spread the fingers of the supporting arm on the floor for balance.

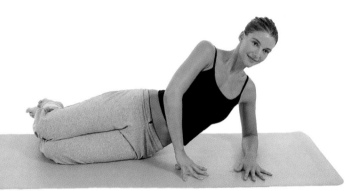

level 1 (just starting out)

- Lie on the floor on your left side and ensure that your knees and hips are stacked in one smooth line.
- Place your elbow underneath your shoulder and relax both shoulder blades. Inhale and prepare.
- Exhale and lift your left hip off the floor while distributing your weight evenly on your elbow and knee. This may be difficult at first so use your right hand to help you balance. Hold this position for 3–5 breaths and release.

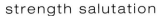

level 3 (strong) – transition

- Lie on your left side as before, ensure your hips and knees are stacked in one smooth line.
- Bend your lower left leg for support and stretch the top right leg long with the foot pointed. Extend your left arm so that you are supporting yourself on your hand this time rather than your elbow.

level 3 – T-stand

- As you exhale pull in your stomach and stretch your right arm to the sky, ensuring that your hips are in line with your knees.
- Imagining you are between two panes of glass, hold yourself in one straight line. Look up towards your right hand. Engage your buttock muscles (gluteals) and extend your right leg. Either keep your top leg extended on the floor or you can lift it slightly to further engage the thigh muscles.

crocodile press

This is a strong upper body exercise designed to tone and sculpt your upper arms and torso. Work through the levels progressively always resting between sets in Child Pose (see page 82). There are three levels for you to choose from. Use the level that feels comfortable to you. You will naturally gravitate to more advanced positions as you adjust to the patterns of movement.

BENEFITS

Strengthens and tones the upper torso and the backs of your upper arms, which helps lifting and pushing tasks. Also improves muscle tone.

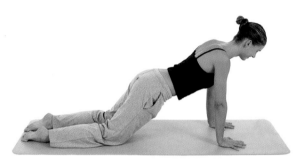

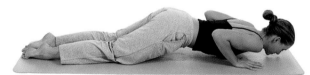

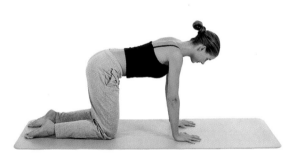

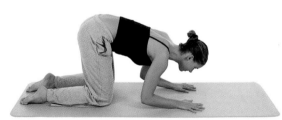

level 2 (getting stronger)

- Again, on all fours, come into the three-quarter position by shifting your hips in front of your knees. Pull your belly in towards your spine.
- Position your hands beneath your shoulders and keep your shoulders relaxed.
- Breathe in to prepare your body for the exhalation, pressing the weight of your torso towards the floor. Keep your elbows locked inwards. Keep your neck in line with the rest of your spine.
- Breathe out as you lower yourself towards the floor and release any tension.
- Breathe in as you push back up to the starting position and repeat 8, 10 or 12 times.

level 1 (just starting out)

- Start by kneeling on all fours. Make sure your hips and knees are in a straight line, and that your shoulders and hands are also aligned.
- Spread your fingers on the floor to take your weight evenly and relax your feet.
- Inhale and prepare. As you exhale press your torso down towards the floor. Take care to keep your elbows locked in line with your waist to isolate the triceps muscles.
- Inhale and push back up to the starting position. Repeat 8, 10 or 12 times.

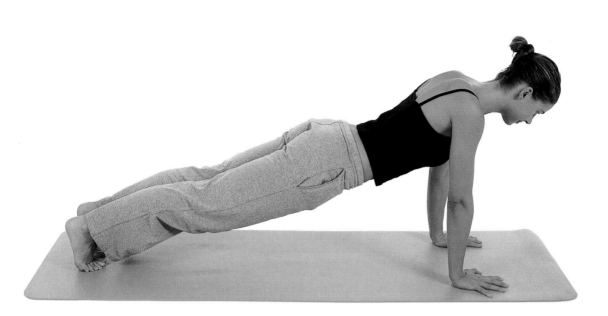

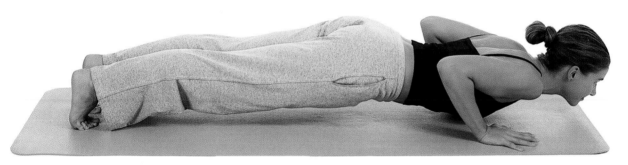

level 3 (strong)

- From the initial all-fours position, extend both legs out behind you, one at a time, to come into the Long-Arm Plank position, similar to the press-up position but with your hands only shoulder width apart.
- Contract your thighs by lifting your kneecaps. Keep your legs contracted and your buttocks switched on to provide a strong base. Keep your chest open.
- Spread your fingers on the floor to take your weight evenly. Pull your stomach in to protect the spine.
- Inhale and prepare. As you slowly exhale, lower your torso to a comfortable range from the floor. Keep your elbows tightly into your waist. Ensure the core abdominals stay strong.
- Any dipping through the hips indicates a weakness in the posture and you should revert back to level 2 to remedy this.
- Inhale and push back up to the starting position. Repeat 8, 10 or 12 times.

rocker

The Rocker is a dynamic movement designed to ease tension through the rolling motion whilst strengthening and toning the abdominals and back extensors.

BENEFITS
Works the abdominals and back extensors in a functional manner to improve core strength for everyday living. Improves posture.

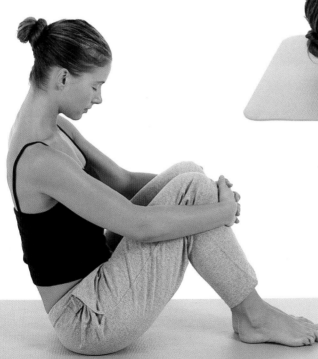

2 lift feet
• Inhale then lift both feet off the floor, relaxing your shoulders behind you. Pull in through the core to make the muscles work.

1 starting position
• Sit on the end of your mat. Tuck your chin into your chest and keep your feet flat on the floor. Round the spine so that you can rock smoothly.

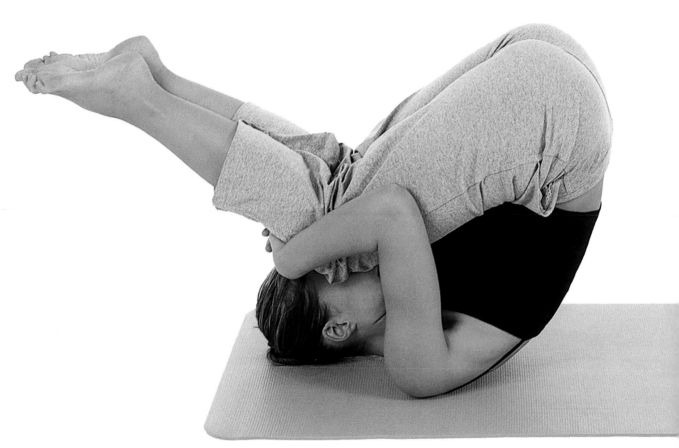

3 rock backwards

- On the same inhale rock backwards. Keep your knees hugged into your chest and make sure your chin is tucked in. Do not roll on to your neck.
- Exhale as you rock back up to the seated position. Pull through the strength in your abdominals to sit up.

Levels of difficulty

Step 4 offers three levels for you to
choose from. Use the level that feels
comfortable to you. You will naturally
gravitate to more advanced positions as
you adjust to the patterns of movement.

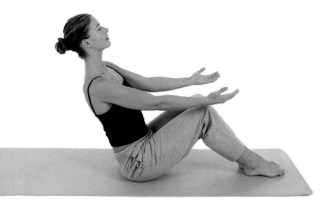

4 level 1 (just starting out)

- Rock back up to a V–Sit Stabilizer position (see
  page 64). Exhale, and ensure there is no bulging
  out of your abdominals. Hold for 1 breath.
- Raise your arms to shoulder level, your palms
  facing upwards to the sky to catch the energy. Lift
  your chest and relax your shoulders while gently
  pulling in the 'B' line (bikini/belt line).
- Look up to an imaginary sun, which is slightly
  above and in front of you.

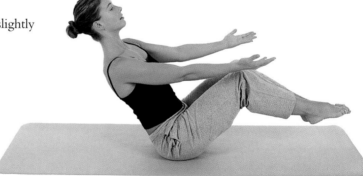

4 level 2 (getting stronger)

- Begin as for Level 1, but this time come out of
  the rocking motion on your exhale and pull on
  the abdominals to stop gravity taking your feet
  all the way to the floor.
- Hold the V–Sit Stabilizer position for 2 breaths,
  inhale and rock back without resting your feet
  on the floor.
- Repeat 8, 10 or 12 times.

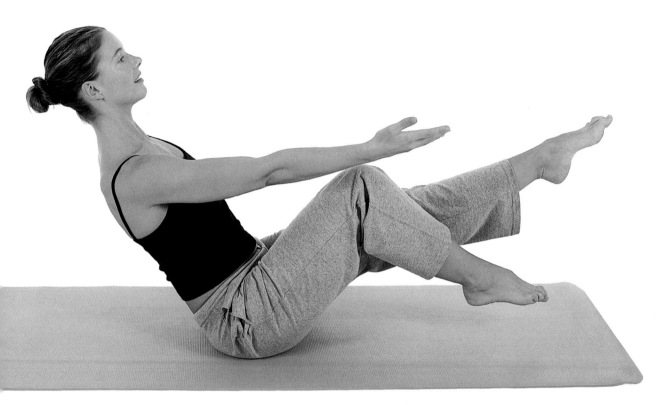

4 level 3 (strong)

- As before, rock backwards while inhaling and exhale as you rock back up again to extend one leg in front of you. This places more emphasis on your abdominals and spine. Make sure the abdominals do not 'dome' during the static hold – this is important for abdominal and spine stabilization.
- Contract the thigh muscle on the extended leg.
- Inhale and repeat the rocking movement with alternate leg extensions each time.

stress-free salutation

shower of light

This exercise draws in fresh *chi* to recharge you and for cleanses harmful *chi* from the energy field that surrounds you. A shower of light washes over you, washing away all the stagnant *chi* and bathing the body with fresh *chi*.

BENEFITS
Enhances mental concentration, relaxes the nervous system and helps eliminate stress.

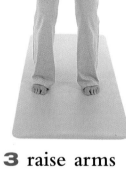

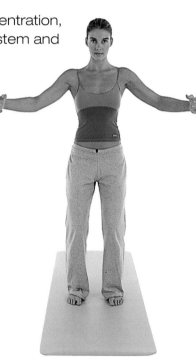

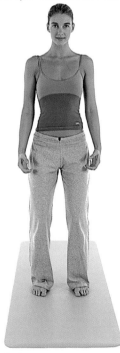

3 raise arms
• Continue raising your arms up above your head. Keep them relaxed and soft at all times to allow the soft and gentle flow of *chi*. Continue inhaling to absorb the energy in the rising motion of the 'shower'.

2 lift arms
• Breathing in, begin to raise your arms upwards.

1 horse stance
• Stand in a horse stance – your legs apart as though astride a horse and your knees soft. Ensure your whole body is relaxed.
• Have your arms at your sides, palms facing your thighs. Pull your navel into your spine, and lengthen your spine upwards.

> 'imagine fresh energy
> filling your palms
> from the sun above'

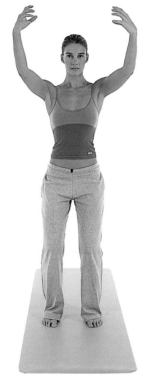

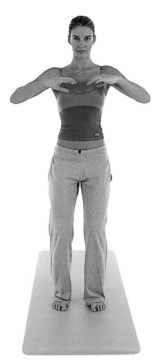

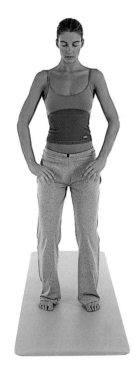

4 absorb energy

- When your arms are above your body imagine fresh energy filling your palms from the sun above. Imagine you have sponge gloves on your hands and all the energy is being absorbed into the palms of your hands.
- Exhale and release your arms down over the top of your head in front of your face.

5 clear the *chi*

- Bring the energy into your body and down past your face, chest and belly. As you do this imagine the new energy sweeping down your body, gathering and clearing away all the stagnant *chi*. Keep your palms facing into your body as you sweep downwards.

6 closing

- Continue to exhale and gently drop your jaw as your hands softly move down to finish the breath.

sink the *chi*

This exercise focuses your mind into your breath and becoming aware of any chest tension or anxiety you may be carrying. Repeat as many times as necessary to recharge your energy levels and focus the breath into the mind rather than your stresses or pressure. Start with 5 minutes of breathing in this way every day and slowly work up to 10 minutes if you can.

BENEFITS
Improves your ability to diffuse toxins out of the body via the exhalation. Seals fresh energy into your body.

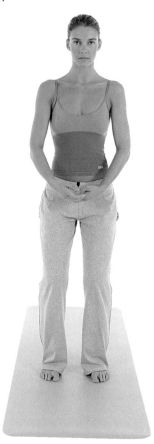

2 initiate the breath

- Inhale gently, bring your hands together and prepare to lift your arms out to the sides like a peacock showing its beautiful colours. Bend your knees slightly as you begin to breathe.

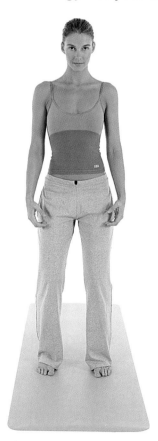

1 horse stance

- Stand in a horse stance – your legs apart as though astride a horse and your knees soft. Ensure your shoulders are relaxed.

'lift your arms out to the sides like a peacock showing its beautiful colours'

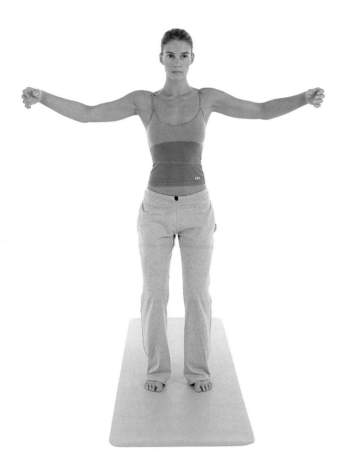

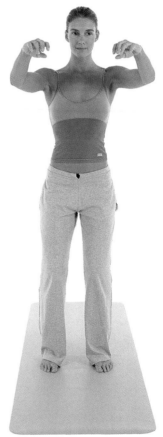

3 lift arms sideways

• Keep inhaling and gently lift your arms to the sides, making sure that you keep your hands soft and relaxed.

4 begin to sink the *chi*

• Keep inhaling and bring your hands all the way in front of you as if gathering the entire positive *chi* from the inhale. Draw your hands in towards your chest.

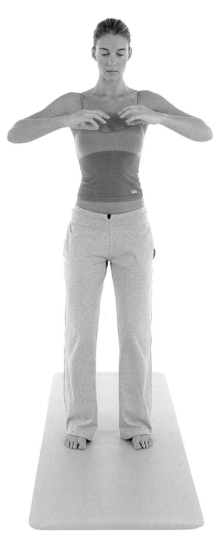

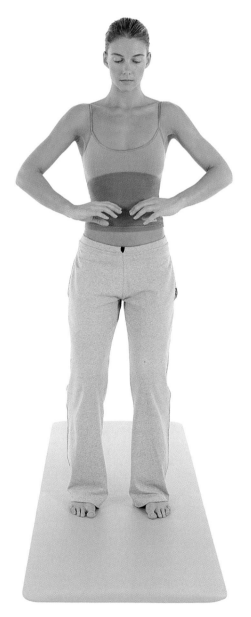

'imagine clearing the breath of all blockages'

5 sink the high *chi*
- As your hands come close to your chest, gently turn your palms down to face the floor and begin to exhale out the entire stagnant *chi*. Imagine clearing the breath of all blockages.

6 sink the middle *chi*
- Keep exhaling gently while guiding your hands down to the lower abdomen area.

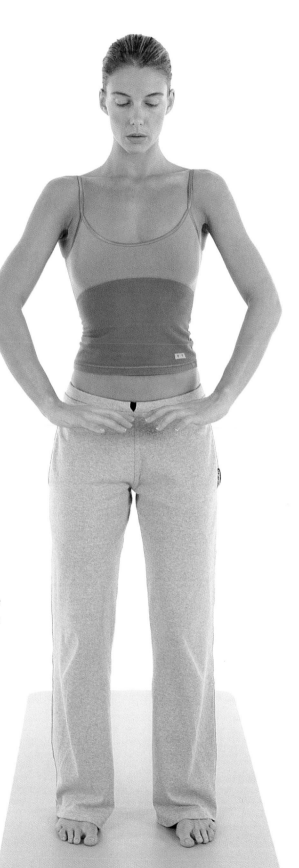

7 sink the lower *chi*

- Keep exhaling slowly, guide your breath with the physical hand movement. Imagine pushing down a float in water and work gently against the resistance with your breath.
- If you find it difficult to hold on to the breath, do not strain. Instead, just gently take another breath to help you.

scapular push-ups

This is a great destressing exercise for shoulder and neck tension. Perform the exercise 8–12 times for a minimum of 2–4 sets with rests in between. There are three levels for you to choose from. Use the level that feels comfortable to you. You will naturally gravitate to more advanced positions as you adjust to the patterns of movement. Anyone with any back problems should stay low on scapular push-ups and stick with Level 1.

BENEFITS
Improves posture and releases the shoulder and uper back of tension or pain. Relieves headaches or neck pain.

level 1 (just getting started)

- Lie face down on the floor. Imagining there is a drawing pin or a piece of holly beneath your belly button, pull your belly in towards your spine and away from your mat.
- Inhale and lift your chest up off the floor, taking care to keep your head in alignment with the rest of your spine. Keep your elbows on the floor for extra support.
- Exhale when in position.
- Inhale and elevate your shoulders to your ears. Imagine your ears and shoulders are joined together.
- Exhale and release shoulder blades down and away from ear lobes once more.

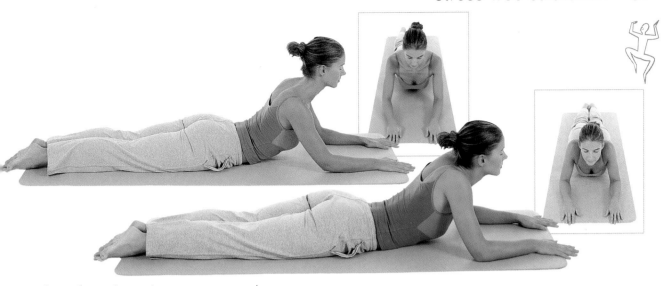

level 2 (getting stronger)

• As long as you have no known spine condition and you have strong back muscles, you can progress to Level 2. Inhale and hollow out your belly. Lift your torso up higher off the floor so that your elbows are closer together.

• Keep your chest open and your head in neutral. Exhale when in position.

• Inhale and elevate your shoulders to your ears. Imagine you have Velcro on your ears and shoulders, joining them together.

• Exhale and release shoulder blades down and away from ear lobes.

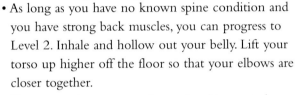

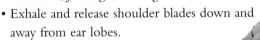

level 3 (strong)

• Exhale and engage the muscles attached to your shoulder blades (the scapular muscles), drawing your shoulder blades down your back towards the pelvis and creating as much space between your shoulders and ears as possible.

• Inhale and elevate your shoulders then exhale and draw the blades away. Repeat 8, 10 or 12 times as desired, breathing deeply throughout for a minimum of 2 sets.

child pose

This is a great exercise for anybody who sits for long periods of time as the curling posture releases any tension in the spine. Hold for 3–5 long breaths or for as long as desired. If you have problems with your knees, go back only as far as is comfortable or sit back on a cushion.

BENEFITS

Allows the intervertebral discs to rehydrate thus protecting the spine from compression or back ache. Lengthens the spine and releases back discomfort.

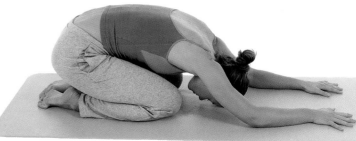

2 sit back

• Inhale and prepare, then exhale and ease your buttocks on to your heels. Lean forwards until your head touches the ground, stretching your arms along the ground in front of you. Feel a comfortable stretch in the lower spine and relax your shoulders. Ensure that your belly is hollowed so as to support the spine.

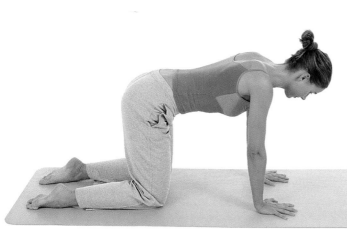

1 start position

• Kneeling on all fours, pull the 'B' line (bikini/belt line) in towards your spine. Keep your head in line with the rest of the spine.

• Ensure all your fingers are spread evenly to share the weight of your torso with the heels of your hands and your wrists. The tops of your feet should be relaxed on the floor.

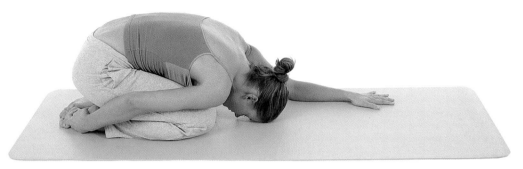

3 tuck arms away

- Release one arm behind you and relax the back of the hand on the ground, the palm facing upwards to absorb energy. Allow the fingers to relax and cup. This allows the shoulder to relax and frees it from the elevation and tension experienced at stressful times.

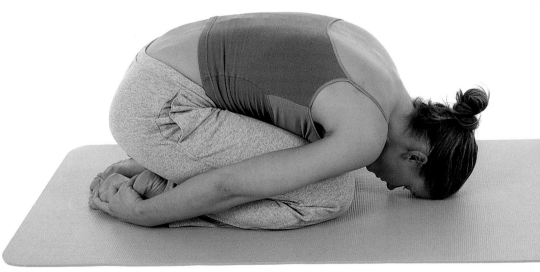

4 child pose

- Release the other arm behind you and relax this hand in the same way. Stay like this for 3–5 breaths or as long as is comfortable.
- Use your breathing to help your body sink further into this pose and release tension from your spine, thighs, hips and possibly your calves. The deeper you breathe in and out the lower you will go.

regeneration

This posture may seem simple but switching the mind into your own unique breathing patterns is in fact a fine skill. It will help you focus the mind inwards on yourself rather than on others or on demands being placed upon you. This is your meditation period, which ideally should be done daily, and can last for 5–15 minutes.

Try regeneration at least once a day. If you have trouble connecting your mind and body you are shifting more thoughts than is healthy for you.

BENEFITS
Mental rest, rejuvenates the nervous system, adrenal glands and thyroid. Aids deep sleep and vital cell renewal.

relaxation

❖ Lie on your back on the floor, making sure that you are warm.

❖ Relax your whole body, checking that your spine is straight and your head and neck are released from tension. Let your limbs fall open each side of your spine, while your toes fall outwards and your palms face upwards.

❖ Close your eyes, and allow them to soften. Take a deep breath in. As you exhale allow your body to drop into the mat. Become aware of your whole body and notice any little sensations you feel. With every exhalation your body should feel heavier.

pause...

❖ As you begin to relax, allow a short positive affirmation to form in your mind, for example 'I am getting better and better every single day in every single way'.

pause...

❖ Repeat it gently to yourself, three times, with meaning. You are in control. The reins to your own body are in your own hands, so enjoy the ride – no one else can. You are your very own unique and amazing human being.

pause...

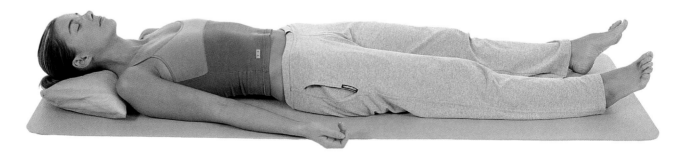

❧ As you relax, bring your awareness into the following parts of the body, pausing between each and scanning them visually in your mind. See it happen. See your body and mind as you want them to be...

❧ Become aware of the palm of your right hand... the back of your hand... your wrist... your forearm... your elbow... your upper arm... your right shoulder... the right side of your waist... the right side of your pelvis... the top of your right leg... your right knee... your right calf... your right ankle... the top of your right foot... the sole of your right foot... your toes.

❧ Now repeat the above instructions on the other side slowly, beginning with the palm of your left hand and saying them to yourself as you reach each part in turn.

pause...

❧ Bring your awareness into the back of your body lying on the floor. Become aware of your right shoulder blade... your left shoulder blade... your right lower back... your left lower back... your right buttock... your left buttock... relax the whole of your back into the ground beneath you... keep relaxed but do not fall asleep.

❧ Take your awareness to the crown of your head. Bring your awareness into your skull... the brow... the right eye... the left eye... the right cheek... the left cheek... the right side of your face... the left side of your face... the throat... the collar bones... Moving your awareness down, relax your collar bones... the right ribs... and left ribs... sink your awareness deep into the belly... the belly button... feed the organs with your slow conscious breath.

❧ Now bring your awareness into your right leg from the hips to the toes... into your left leg from the hips to the toes... Become aware of both legs together... release the length of both legs... release the length of both arms... Become aware of your whole body... calmly relaxing on the floor...

pause...

❧ Now listen to your breath and become aware of the frequency, the ebb and the volume... be aware of the flow of breath entering and exiting your body... with no effort at all... simply awareness... of the breath... washing through your mind and body.

❧ Sink your mind into your core... feel the warmth of your core... feel the core rise on the inhale... and sink on the exhale... Journey with this breath... let it lead you... listen to it... get to know it... love it... breathe it... a soft journey undertaken with the breath.

❧ Now bring your awareness back to the positive statement that you formed at the beginning of the practice. Keep aware, yet deeply relaxed. This is effortless. Form the statement in your mind, and repeat it to yourself three times over clearly with meaning.

❧ Follow the rhythm of each breath... allowing your body to remain completely still. Become aware of your body in contact with the ground... feel your body breathing. Now become aware of the space around you... of the room around you... gently allow your body to expand as you breathe energy into it. Begin to slowly wiggle your fingers and the tips of your toes. Take your time awakening, very slowly...

❧ Begin to stretch deep within your spine... Yawn into your whole body as if awakening from a deep replenishing sleep. When you are ready, roll on to your right side, resting as long as you need to before sitting up. Take your time and stretch as you need to.

pyramid breathing

This is a great way of releasing energy into the spine and pelvic areas. It combines your breath with physical movement using your breathing as your guide. It is best performed after the regeneration exercise. Perform the exercise 5–10 times on each side.

BENEFITS

Recharges the body slowly with energy and awakens the muscles and body for action.

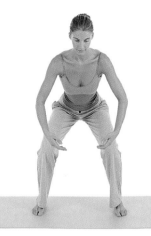

3 initiate body

• Bend through your knees on the inhalation and raise your arms up and out.

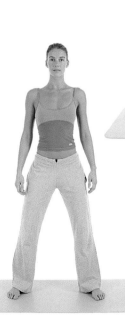

2 initiate breath

• Inhale, and bring your hands in front of you, arms loose and with your palms facing upwards.

1 start position

• Stand with your feet one-and-a-half times your shoulder width apart. Have your hands relaxed at your sides and your chest open and lengthened.

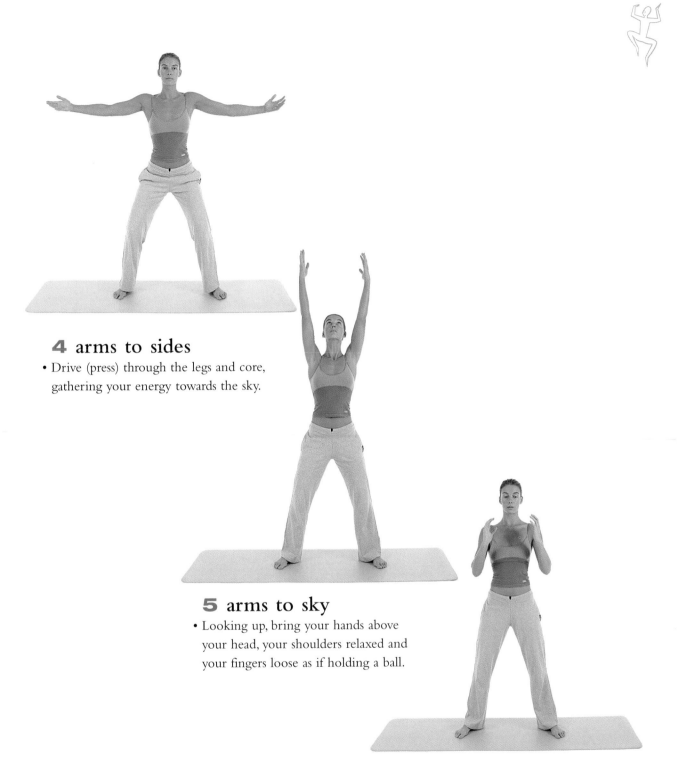

4 arms to sides
• Drive (press) through the legs and core, gathering your energy towards the sky.

5 arms to sky
• Looking up, bring your hands above your head, your shoulders relaxed and your fingers loose as if holding a ball.

6 lower energy
• Exhale and draw your palms down to recharge.

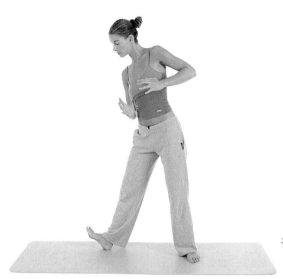

7 turning

• Inhale and turn your right foot
out to the side. Continue
breathing in.

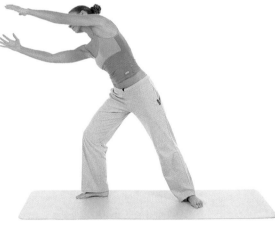

8 drive

• Still inhaling, drive through
the legs and core and move
the ball of energy out towards
the side. Press through your
pelvis and pull your belly in
towards your spine.

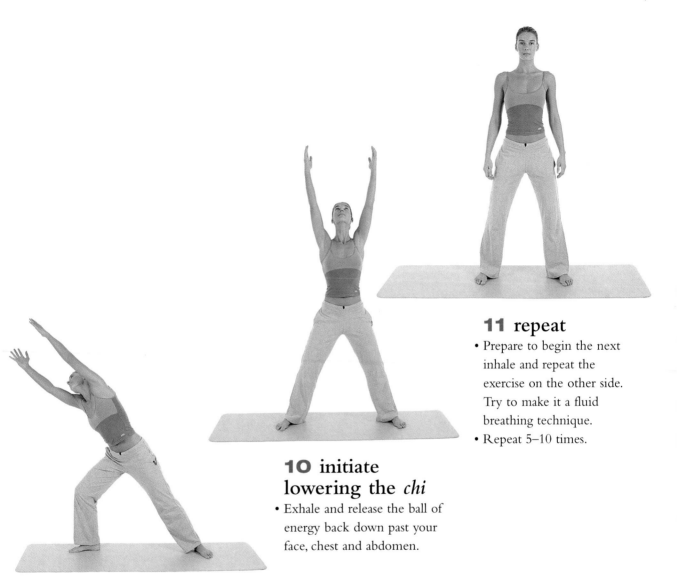

11 repeat
- Prepare to begin the next inhale and repeat the exercise on the other side. Try to make it a fluid breathing technique.
- Repeat 5–10 times.

10 initiate lowering the *chi*
- Exhale and release the ball of energy back down past your face, chest and abdomen.

9 catch the *chi*
- Lift the ball of energy up to the sky using the power through your body core and lower spine. Keep breathing in smoothly.

dusk salutation

BENEFITS
Lengthens the body and switches on the transversus abdominis muscle, which provides true functional core strength and balance for everyday life.

1 neutral alignment

- Stand at the front of the mat with your feet together and your weight spread evenly. Your arms should be hanging loosely by your sides with your palms against your thighs. Spread your toes out on the floor like piano keys and ground the four corners of your feet. Pull your thigh muscles into the bone so that your kneecaps lift.

- Lift your upper body out of the seat of the pelvis, centring your body each side of your spine. Tuck your tailbone down and lengthen your spine upwards keeping the skin on the back of the neck wrinkle-free and smooth. Engage your pelvic floor by 30 per cent. Feel your rib cage floating above your pelvis. Breathe deeply into your side ribs. Widen your collarbones, keeping the shoulders soft, but the armpits lifted.

- Press through the soles of your feet and lift the crown of your head towards the sky. Feel a stretch within your body – from the pelvis down, rooted into the earth, and from your pelvis upwards, lifting your upper body towards the sky. Look straight ahead as if towards an imaginary horizon.

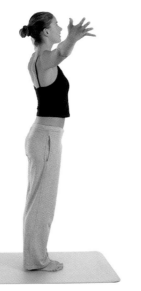

'imagine you
are standing
on the top of
a mountain'

2 transition

- Begin to inhale calmly through your
  nose and lift your arms up and out to
  the sides. Hold on to your core
  connection and keep your pelvis
  tucked slightly.

BENEFITS
Great for breathing
and expanding the
lungs. Gets rid of
all the tension that
pulls our bodies
down throughout
the day.

3 mountain pose

- Inhale through your nose and slowly
  extend your arms up towards the sky.
  Imagine you are standing on the top of
  a mountain and you are breathing in
  lots of fresh *chi* for your body to absorb.

4 transition

- Exhale and release your torso out and
  down towards the floor, your arms
  hanging below your head. Imagine diving
  off your mountain into a beautiful warm
  ocean. Pull your belly in towards your
  spine and keep your feet grounded.

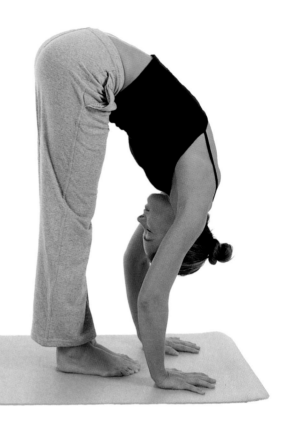

BENEFITS
Releases compression in the lower spine caused by long bouts of sitting or standing and improves blood flow to the upper body. Lengthens the backs of the thighs (hamstrings).

5 standing fold

- Relax in the standing fold for a few breaths to release any compression in the lower spine. Your spine will be released a little further each time you perform this salutation.
- Relax your hands on the floor.

'Do not worry if your hands do not reach the floor. This is your journey and your body will naturally move towards the floor as you practise.'

BENEFITS
Gives you a good indication of your hip mobility and the movement surrounding the lower spine, hips and thighs.

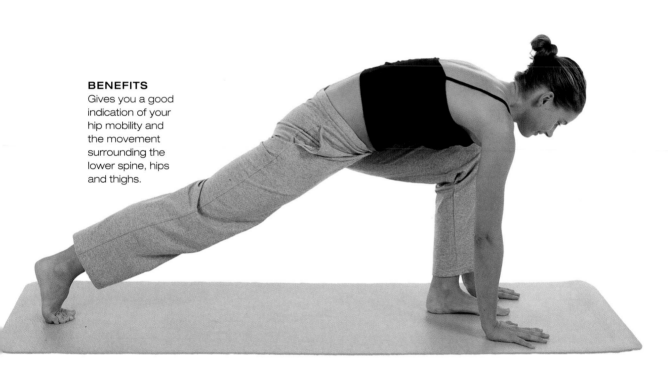

6 step back

- Inhale and step your right leg backwards. Keep your front leg stable by activating the foot muscles and fanning the toes.
- Exhale in this new position and recover.

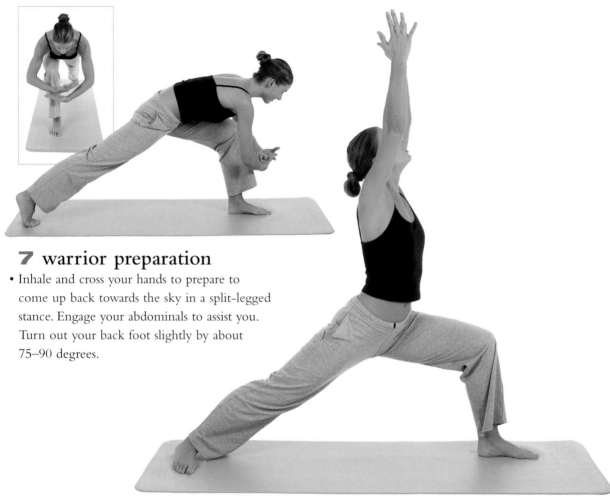

7 warrior preparation

- Inhale and cross your hands to prepare to come up back towards the sky in a split-legged stance. Engage your abdominals to assist you. Turn out your back foot slightly by about 75–90 degrees.

8 split stance preparation

- Keep breathing in the fresh *chi* as you extend upwards. Bring your hands all the way above your shoulders and keep your fingers long and strong. Move your arms outwards as if gathering all the energy and saluting the sun.
- Drive through both legs as you move. Lengthen through your spine like a puppet on a string. Ensure that both your heels are in line.

'move your arms outwards as if gathering all the energy and saluting the sun'

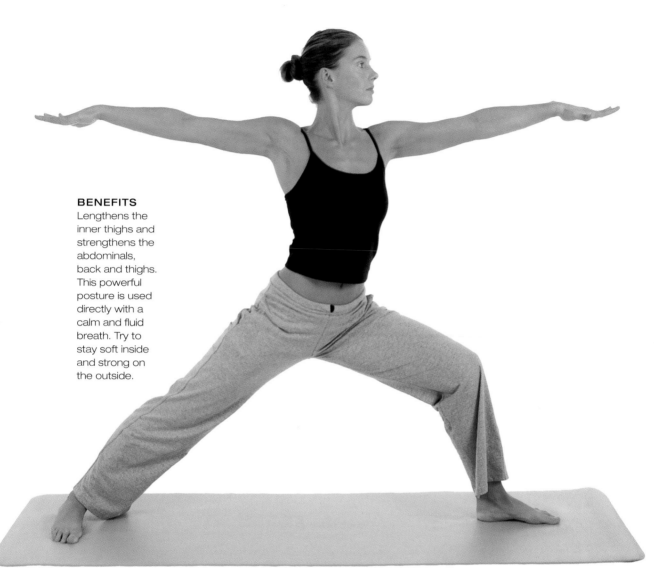

BENEFITS
Lengthens the inner thighs and strengthens the abdominals, back and thighs. This powerful posture is used directly with a calm and fluid breath. Try to stay soft inside and strong on the outside.

9 warrior

- Exhale and lower your left arm in front and the right arm behind. Your fingers should remain long and your palms facing down. Relax your shoulders. Engage your abdominals to support you and keep your shoulders and hips in line.
- Turn your left foot forwards while your back right foot should be at a 45–90-degree angle.
- Breathe in and out 3–5 times, lowering a little further through your legs as you exhale.

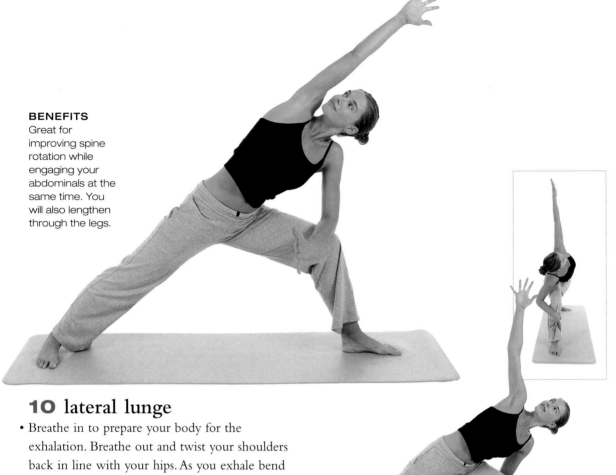

BENEFITS
Great for improving spine rotation while engaging your abdominals at the same time. You will also lengthen through the legs.

10 lateral lunge

- Breathe in to prepare your body for the exhalation. Breathe out and twist your shoulders back in line with your hips. As you exhale bend over to your left and extend your right arm over and above your head, while staying in line with the rest of your body.
- Place your left elbow on the inside of your left thigh for a little support. Pull in your core and keep your hips lifted. Drive through your feet and ensure they are fully grounded. Check that your heels are still in line with each other, on an imaginary tightrope.
- Remain in this position for 3–5 breaths, and as you exhale ease your shoulders and hips further in line.

11 transition

- Inhale and lift up your right arm to create a straight line with your shoulder. Look up at your hand.
- Exhale, place your left hand on your shin and ease your shoulders back to be in line with your hips. This will feel a little more difficult than the lateral lunge as you have extended your hand further down.
- Pull in your abdominals and switch on the thighs to help you drive and breathe further into the posture.

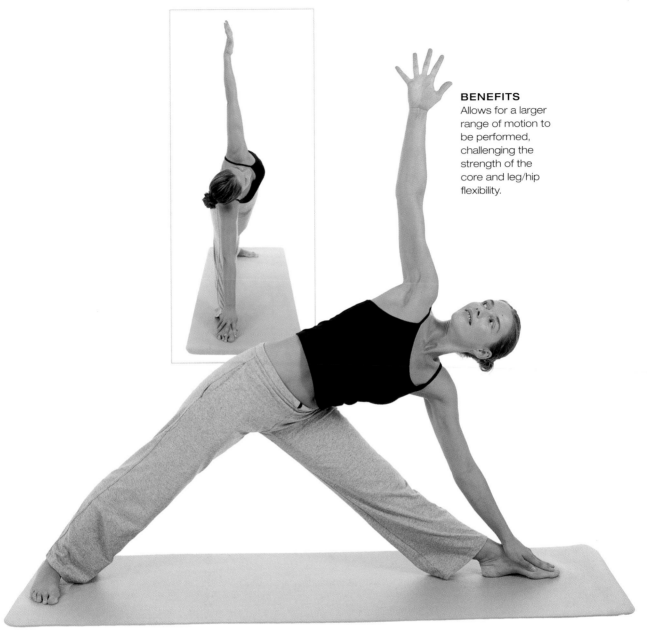

BENEFITS
Allows for a larger range of motion to be performed, challenging the strength of the core and leg/hip flexibility.

12 triangle pose

- If you feel able to take this into the full triangle without losing your shoulder and hip line, inhale and lower your left hand to your ankle.
- Exhale and straighten your front leg so you get a fantastic stretch up the back of the front leg.
- Stay here for 3–5 breaths and breathe your tension away into the atmosphere.

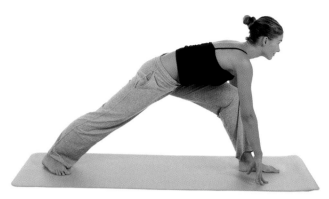

13 transition 1

- Inhale and rotate your torso back to the centre and bring your right arm down. Be careful to breathe into this twist, as your back ankle will still be at an angle.
- Pull the 'B' line (bikini/belt line) inwards and your shoulders away from your ears to keep your back strong.

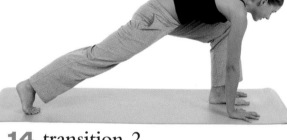

14 transition 2

- Turn your back foot to face forwards – imagine you are standing either side of a train track instead of on a tightrope.
- Exhale in this position to recover.

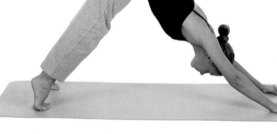

15 transition 3

- Inhale and step your left leg back at hip distance from your right foot so you are in an inverted 'V' position. Lift your heels off the floor and contract the thigh muscles to assist with the stretch in the backs of your legs.
- Pull your belly in toward your spine and retract your shoulder blades behind you, drawing them together like curtains.
- Spread your fingers and ensure your wrists are supported. Your head should be relaxed.

BENEFITS
Builds upper body
strength and lower
body flexibility.
Releases any
tension in the hips.

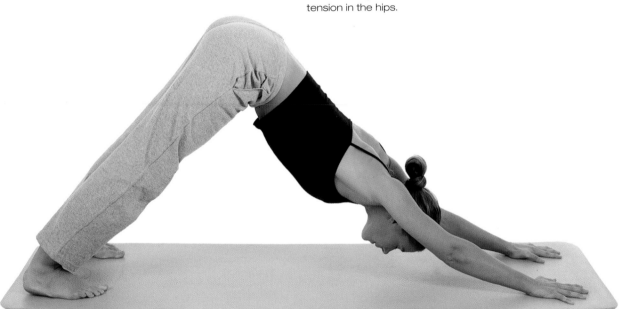

16 downward dog

- Exhale and ease your heels back to the floor.
  Zip in your pelvic floor 30 per cent and hollow
  out the belly to support your spine.
- Draw your shoulder blades from your ears,
  keeping your head relaxed. Hold for 3–5 breaths.
- Fill up with fresh *chi* and elevate your tailbone to
  the sky. Exhale the stagnant *chi* and ease further
  into the downward dog position.

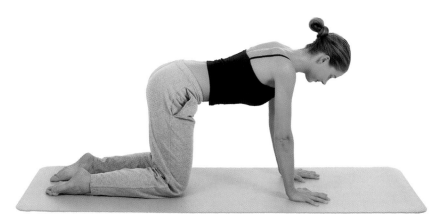

17 transition 1

- Exhale and release both your knees to the floor until you are kneeling on all fours.
- Pull your belly in towards your spine and ensure your shoulders are relaxed and away from your ears. The tops of your feet should be relaxed on the floor.

18 transition 2

- Inhale, move your buttocks back to your heels and as you exhale sink your buttocks behind you. Lean forwards until your head touches the ground, stretching your arms along the ground in front of you. Rest your shoulders and release your right arm away behind you.

BENEFITS
Allows the intervertebral discs to rehydrate and the lower spine to soften and recover.

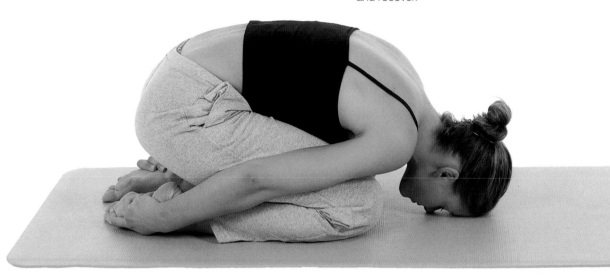

19 child pose

- Release your left arm away behind you, your palms facing upwards. Stay here and focus on pulling your belly in towards your spine.
- Breathe, fill up with fresh *chi*. Release the breath without dropping your back downwards.

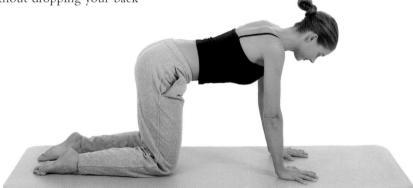

20 transition

- Inhale and push through your fingers and abdomen back on to all fours. Zip in your belly and core.

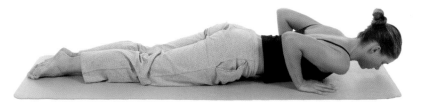

21 transition 1

• Exhale and lower your torso to the floor. Keep
your hands by the sides of your chest. Hollow
out your belly for support.

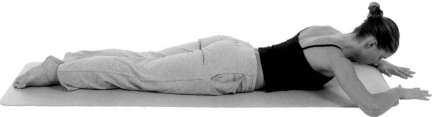

22 transition 2

• Extend your arms halfway in front of your
shoulders. Spread your fingers out on the floor
and relax your elbows at the side.

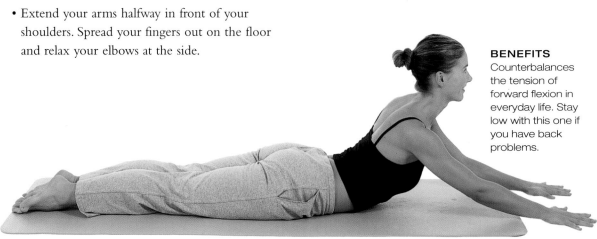

BENEFITS
Counterbalances
the tension of
forward flexion in
everyday life. Stay
low with this one if
you have back
problems.

23 cobra

• Inhale and push through your fingertips and arms
up into the Cobra position. Pull your belly in
towards your spine and away from the mat –
imagine there is a drawing pin or a piece of holly
beneath your belly button, which you do not
want to touch.

• Keeping your shoulders away from your ears and
your hips on the floor, feel a great stretch through
the spine.

'cobra lengthens
the spine and
initiates a
re-energizing
backbend'

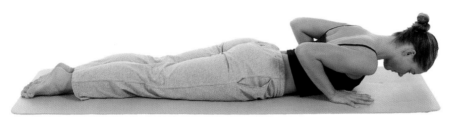

24 transition

- Exhale and lower yourself, drawing your hands back into the sides of your chest. Keep your 'B' line (bikini/belt line) lifted.

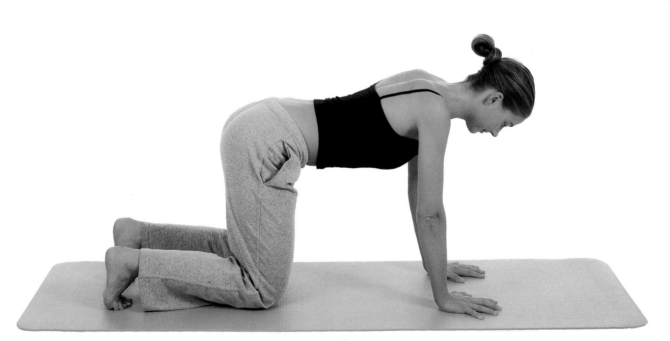

BENEFITS
Allows you to practice keeping neutral alignment in a box position before moving to harder poses.

25 box

- Inhale and push up to an all-fours position, zipping in your abdominals. Curl your feet underneath behind you and exhale.

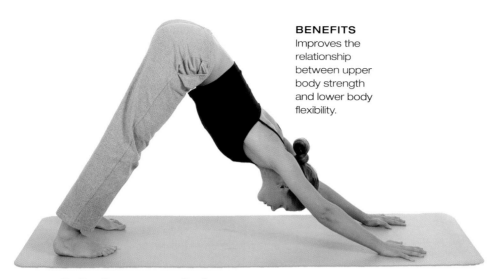

BENEFITS
Improves the relationship between upper body strength and lower body flexibility.

26 downward dog

- Inhale again and drive through the abdomen and legs to extend your tailbone to the sky.
- Draw your shoulder blades together behind you like drawing curtains.
- Contract your thighs to facilitate the stretch up the backs of the legs.
- Exhale and ease your heels down towards the floor to feel a nice stretch up the backs of your legs.

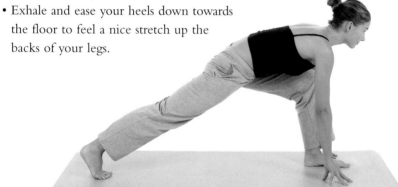

27 transition 1

- Inhale and step your left leg towards your hands. Exhale and pull your belly in towards your spine.
- Look forwards and slightly ahead to keep your chest lifted.

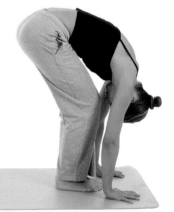

28 transition 2

- Inhale and step your right leg in towards your hands. Exhale and zip in your abdominals. Contract through the muscles in your buttocks (gluteals) and thighs to facilitate the transition.

BENEFITS
Releases
compression in
the lower spine
caused by long
bouts of sitting or
standing and
improves blood
flow to the upper
body. Lengthens
the backs of
the thighs
(hamstrings).

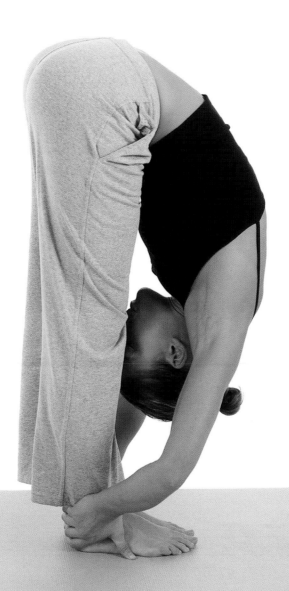

29 standing fold

- Inhale and ease your chest down towards your thighs. You can ease your fold downwards by grounding your hands on the floor or by grasping the backs of your ankles/calves to gently ease yourself lower.
- Exhale and release to recover. Repeat power breaths 3–5 times until you feel you have progressed a little.

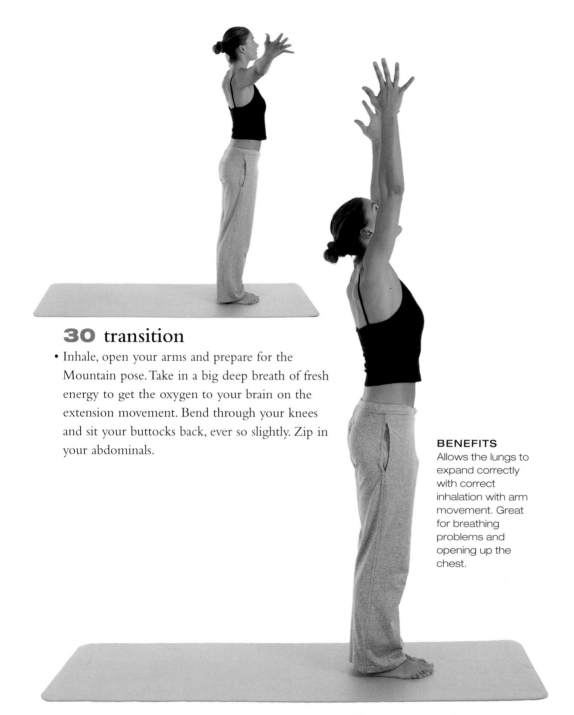

30 transition

- Inhale, open your arms and prepare for the Mountain pose. Take in a big deep breath of fresh energy to get the oxygen to your brain on the extension movement. Bend through your knees and sit your buttocks back, ever so slightly. Zip in your abdominals.

BENEFITS
Allows the lungs to expand correctly with correct inhalation with arm movement. Great for breathing problems and opening up the chest.

31 mountain pose

- Keep inhaling and opening your arms to the sides, raising them until they meet, palms together, at the top.
- Zip up through your chest as well as your abdomen. Lift through the arches in your feet. Contract and engage the legs long and strong.

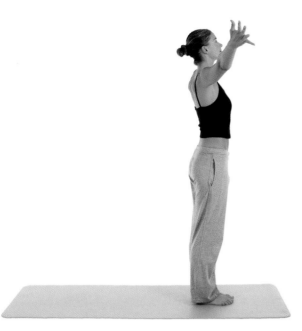

32 transition
- Exhale and release your arms back down to your thighs.

33 neutral alignment
- Exhale and release your arms down to the sides, your palms against your thighs and your neck relaxed in the centre of your shoulder girdle.
- Imagine putting on a belt and breathing in so as to accommodate the innermost notch. Then release your imaginary belt a few notches so that the waist is kept small and the abdominals engaged but the position is comfortable enough to hold with effort.
- Press through the soles of your feet and lift the crown of your head towards the sky. Feel the stretch within your body – from the pelvis down, rooted into the earth, and from your pelvis upwards, lifting your upper body towards the sky. Look straight ahead as if towards an imaginary horizon.

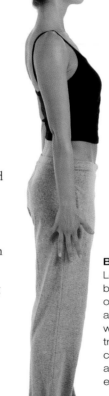

BENEFITS
Lengthens the body and switches on the transversus abdominis muscle, which provides true functional core strength and balance for everyday life.

Levels of difficulty

Steps 34–37 offer four levels of difficulty. Start with step 34 and you will naturally gravitate to the more advanced positions as you adjust to the patterns of movement.

Note: On all levels, your body should be upright. If you are leaning forwards excessively, you should go back to an easier level.

BENEFITS
Encourages good balance and core strength.

34 standing boat pose level 1

- Pull your belly in towards your spine and breathe in to prepare your body for the exhalation.
- As you breathe out lift your right knee until it is level with your hip and point the toe.
- Take both hands around to clasp the knee and pull your scapular blades back to assist a good standing posture.
- Hold for 3–5 breaths.

BENEFITS
By taking the arms away, we challenge the balance further.

35 standing boat pose level 2

- Inhale and lift torso higher.
- Exhale and take arms to the sides.
- Hold for 3–5 breaths.

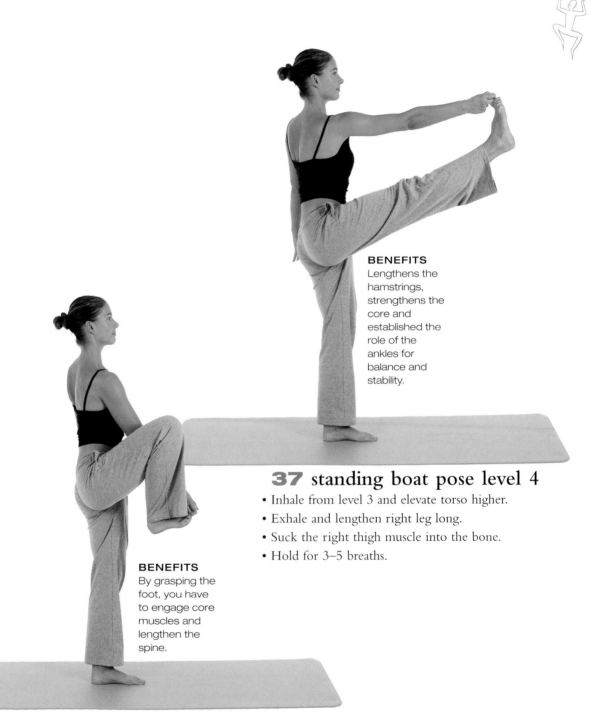

BENEFITS
Lengthens the
hamstrings,
strengthens the
core and
established the
role of the
ankles for
balance and
stability.

BENEFITS
By grasping the
foot, you have
to engage core
muscles and
lengthen the
spine.

37 standing boat pose level 4
- Inhale from level 3 and elevate torso higher.
- Exhale and lengthen right leg long.
- Suck the right thigh muscle into the bone.
- Hold for 3–5 breaths.

36 standing boat pose level 3
- Inhale and lift torso higher.
- Exhale and take a grip of the right big toe with your
  thumb and first two fingers.
- Inhale and prepare the breath.
- Exhale, stand tall and hold for 3–5 breaths.

synergize™ for aches and pains

back basics (see pages 112–119)

The key to maintaining a healthy back lies not only in correct exercise but also in good movement practice and posture all the time, no matter what you are doing. Many causes of back pain are not eased by exercise. We therefore cannot stress strongly enough that you must seek medical advice before you embark on any exercise regime, including Synergize™. Poor posture, muscle imbalances and misuse resulting in faulty movement patterns cause the majority of back problems. Synergize™ exercises are perfect for these cases. You should stop instantly if any movement gives you pain.

❖ These exercises will help prevent back pain and may be suitable in treating back issues.
❖ Learn how to stabilize your neutral alignment (see page 35) first and do not move out of it until you are strong at holding it.
❖ If you have any reason to doubt the condition of your back, do not add rotation (twisting) or flexion (bending) exercises without advice from a consultant.

pmt prevention (see pages 120–125)

This section helps to balance the funtion of the adrenal, thyroid and parathyroid glands by carefully controlling the subtle energy of the breath. These exercises are effective in helping with premenstrual tension and hormone regulation prior to, or during, your period. The exercises are best done together in a routine, alternating from one to the other.

❖ These exercises will help if you suffer from PMT or want to relieve the symptoms.
❖ Balances the adrenal glands, which helps to stabilize hormones.
❖ Relaxes the thyroid and parathyroid to release anxiety and stress.

The easy-to-use exercises and movements in this section will optimize your performance in everyday life and may be the answer to any aches and pains.

immune
boosters (see pages 126–135)

With Synergize™ you have an exercise regime for your mind and body, whatever stage of life you may be in. When you learn to listen to what your body is telling you, you will learn to know which exercises will naturally help you to achieve your goals. Sometimes, if you have had a particularly hectic day, the last thing you will feel like doing is your salutations and this is where the following immune-booster exercises will come in useful. If you do feel-good exercises correctly with the breathing techniques, you will feel the change in energy almost immediately.

❖ Use these exercises whenever you feel your energy is low or when you may be coming down with a cold or other illness.
❖ Strengthen your immune system by enhancing your cell renewal.

headache
solutions (see pages 136–141)

There are hundreds of reasons why we get headaches. Synergize™ is most successful in the prevention and treatment of tension headaches, especially where poor posture is a contributory factor. While dealing with the pressure of everyday life we may be unaware of how tension in the back can creep up towards the neck and sometimes affects the tension within the jaw. Through sitting for long periods of time this tension can pass unnoticed until a headache appears.

❖ These exercises will help you to understand the relationships between the head and the neck.
❖ Learn how to relax by engaging the muscles that set the shoulder blades down into the back.
❖ Release any energy blocks by putting pressure on the meridian energy points that lie on the bones situated around the eyes.

back basics

child pose

Hold for 3–5 long breaths or for as long as desired. If you have problems with your knees, go back only as far as is comfortable or sit back on a cushion.

BENEFITS
Lengthens the spine and releases back discomfort.

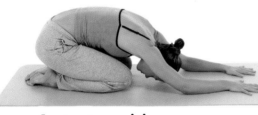

1 start position

- Kneeling on all fours, pull the 'B' line (bikini/belt line) in towards your spine. Keep your head in line with the rest of the spine.
- Ensure all your fingers are spread evenly to share the weight of your torso with the heels of your hands and your wrists. The tops of your feet should be relaxed on the floor.
- Breathe in to prepare your body for the exhalation then breathe out and ease your buttocks on to your heels. Lean forwards until your head touches the ground, stretching your arms along the ground in front of you. Feel a comfortable stretch in the lower spine and relax your shoulders. Ensure that your belly is hollowed so as to support the spine.

2 release arm

- Release one arm behind you and relax the back of the hand on the ground, the palm facing upwards to absorb energy. Allow the fingers to relax and cup. This allows the shoulder to relax and frees it from the elevation and tension experienced particularly at stressful times.

3 child pose

- Release the other arm behind you and relax this hand in the same way. Stay like this for as long as is comfortable.
- Use your breathing to help your body sink further into this pose and release tension from your spine, thighs, hips and possibly your calves. The deeper you breathe in and out the lower you will be able to go.

starfish

The Starfish helps you to coordinate your arms with the opposite legs. Do not be tempted to skip this exercise, as it is crucial in mastering the more difficult exercises on pages 114–119.

BENEFITS
Helps your mind and muscles work more smoothly, while maintaining a neutral spine with moving levers (arms and legs).

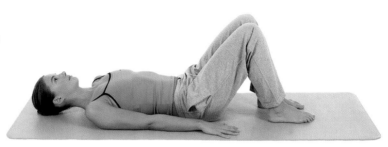

1 start position
- Lie on your back with your legs bent and your feet flat on the floor. Your head should be relaxed and centred, your palms face down on the floor beside your thighs.

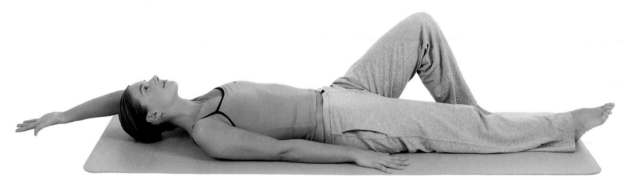

2 starfish position
- Breathe in and fill your lungs. Breathe out, zip in and hollow your core and slide your right leg away from you, along the floor and take your left arm beyond your head in a movement resembling backstroke swimming.
- Keep your pelvis centred and try to limit any rocking from your hips. Keep an open chest and hollowed stomach. Try to keep your shoulder blades away from your ears.
- Breath in, still zipped, and return all of your limbs to the starting position.
- Repeat 5–10 times, alternating the positions of your arms and legs.

toe taps

Toe taps strengthen the abdominals with the synergy of the back muscles to provide protection for your spine through testing everyday activities. Repeat 8–12 times each side, always breathing out on the exertion of lowering your leg.

BENEFITS
Strengthens abdominals and protects the spine.

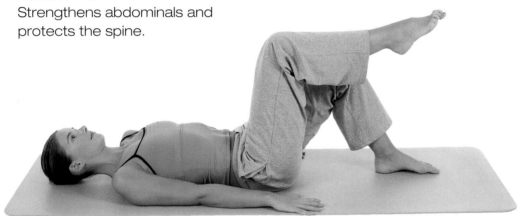

1 lift one leg

- Lie on your back with your legs bent and your feet flat on the floor. Zip in and hollow your belly to provide internal muscular strength around the back and abdominals like an internal corset of support around your middle. Keep your neck long and relaxed and have your palms face down on the floor beside your thighs.
- Inhale and prepare, then exhale, lifting your right leg off the floor at a 90-degree angle.

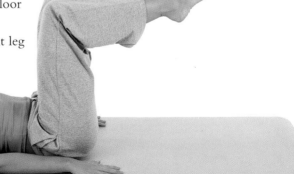

2 lift both legs

- Inhale and prepare. Exhale, staying zipped at the core and lift your left leg to align with the right leg at the same angle. Ensure that your abdominals are still strong.

Levels of difficulty
Steps 3 offer
two levels of difficulty.
Start with level 1
and you will naturally
gravitate to level 2
as you adjust to the
patterns of movement.

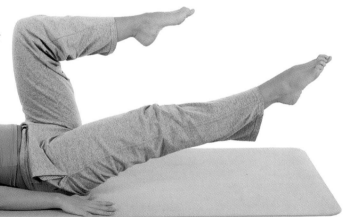

3 level 1 (just starting out)
- Breathe in and prepare. Breathe out on the
  exertion as you slowly lower your right foot, with
  pointed toes, to the floor, as though dipping your
  toe into a pool of warm water.
- Stay zipped in at all times. If you find this
  movement too challenging, keep one leg on
  the floor and simply raise and lower the other
  leg, one at a time, as you breathe out.

3 level 2 (getting stronger)
- Breathe out and extend your right leg while
  bringing the left knee in towards your chest.
  Inhale to recover, exhale and change legs.
  Extending the angle at the knee as you lower
  your leg, thereby creating a longer lever, will
  make this exercise more challenging.
- Repeat 8–12 times each side, always breathing
  out on the exertion of lowering your leg.

table top quadrants

This exercise is very useful for strengthening your back and abdominals while training the smooth synergy of the upper and lower body quadrants. Steps 3–5 offer three levels of difficulty. Start with step 3 and you will naturally gravitate to the more advanced positions as you adjust to the patterns of movement. Perform the exercise 8–12 times for a minimum of 2–4 sets with rests in between.

BENEFITS
Strengthens the shoulders, tones the abdominals and lengthens the spine.

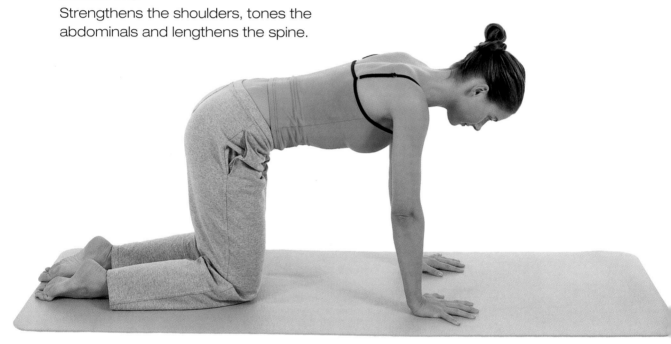

1 starting position

• Start by kneeling on all fours in a 'box' position. Have your hands beneath your shoulders and your hips directly above your knees. Zip in your abdominals. Make sure your shoulder muscles are engaged and drawn away from the ears. Spread your weight evenly through your fingers as well as the heels of your hands.

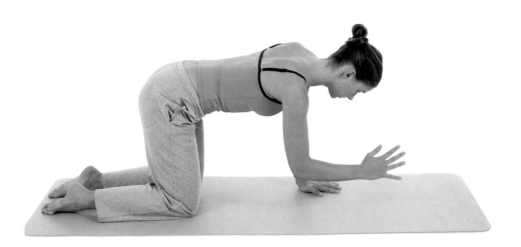

2 transition

- Inhale and prepare. On the exhale slowly lift your right arm up as if reaching for something in front of you. Keeping the neck long and wrinkle-free, tighten through your core and imagine keeping your waist small.

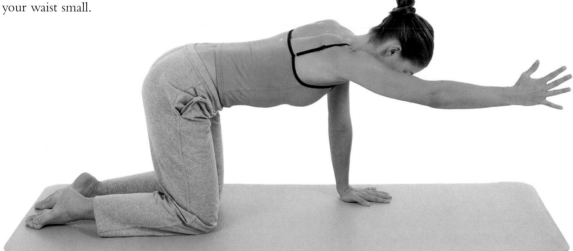

3 level 1 (just starting out)

- Lift your arm in line with your shoulder joint and keep your neck in line with the rest of your spine. Feel the engagement in your shoulders – try to work against gravity and pull your shoulders away from your ears while the arm stays long.
- Breathe in and return your right arm to the start position. Breathe out and repeat the lifts with the other arm.
- Repeat 8–12 times each side.

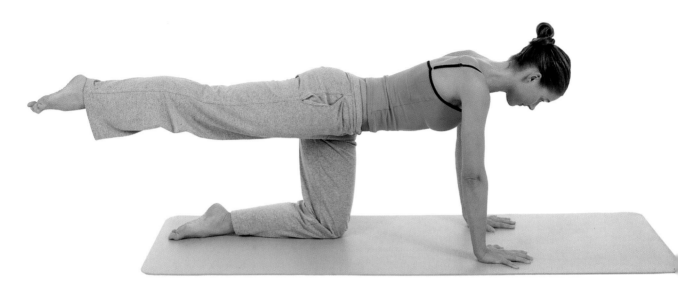

3 level 2 (getting stronger)

- Inhale and prepare your breath in the box start position as at the end of Level 1.
- As you exhale, lift your right leg out, stretching it behind you and engaging the abdominals and spine extensors and buttock muscles. Keep your foot pointed to extend your leg and contract the thigh, which provides more active conditioning.
- Repeat 5–10 times each side.

'suck your thigh muscles into your bones'

'imagine your body having no trouble supporting a very heavy person sitting on your back'

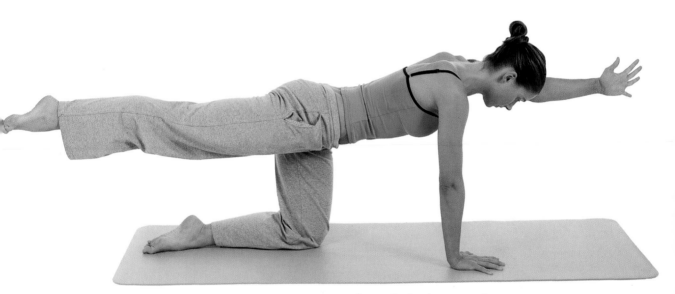

3 level 3 (strong)

- Inhale and prepare your breath in the box start position as at the end of Level 1.
- As you exhale, lift and extend your left arm and right leg at the same time. Suck in your abdominals and imagine your body having no trouble supporting a very heavy person sitting on your back while performing the movement.
- Inhale and return your arm and leg to the box start position. This movement uses the upper and lower quadrants of the body at the same time.
- Repeat the movement, alternating sides, 8–12 times.

pmt prevention
hormone regulation breathing

This exercise regulates the function of the adrenal glands, thyroid and parathyroid by carefully controlling the flow of *chi* by training the breath.

BENEFITS
Calms the nervous system, lowers blood pressure and balances hormone regulation.

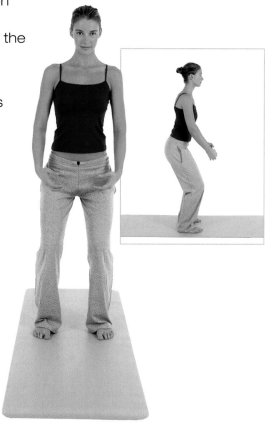

2 initiate breathing

- Take a deep calm breath in while bending through your knees and softening your hips and thighs. Raise your palms to the sky as you breathe.

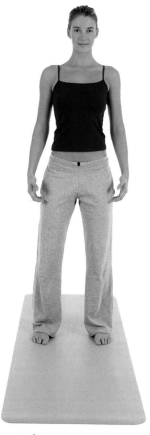

1 horse stance

- Stand in a horse stance – your legs apart as though astride a horse and your knees soft.

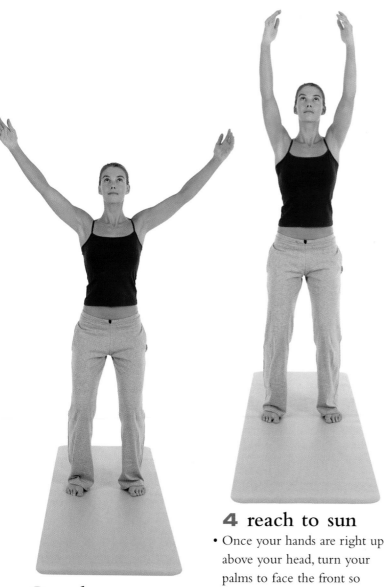

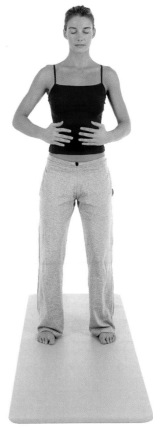

3 gather energy

- Continue to inhale, raising your arms up above your head and slightly in front of you. Slowly turn your palms to face one another.

4 reach to sun

- Once your hands are right up above your head, turn your palms to face the front so that when you lower your arms they can push the *chi* back to the earth.

5 closing

- Bring your hands back down in front of you to your sides as you return back to your heels. Allow your arms to swing down, keeping a natural fluid movement pattern.
- Repeat the exercise 5–10 times before building up to 15–20. You will build a faster rhythm as you become more used to the breathing and physical thread of the movement.

self-lumbar massage

This is a great comforting exercise, which massages the lower spine when experiencing PMT or during your period.

BENEFITS

Stimulates the liver, pancreas and kidneys to promote the removal of toxins.

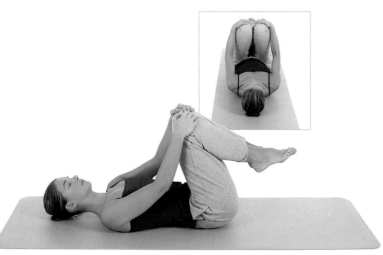

1 start position

• Lie flat on your back, relaxed, with your legs slightly apart and rolling outwards, your arms straight but relaxed, your palms facing upwards. Zip in your abdominals and hollow out your belly. Bring your knees towards your chest so that they are over your hips and hold them to your chest with your hands.

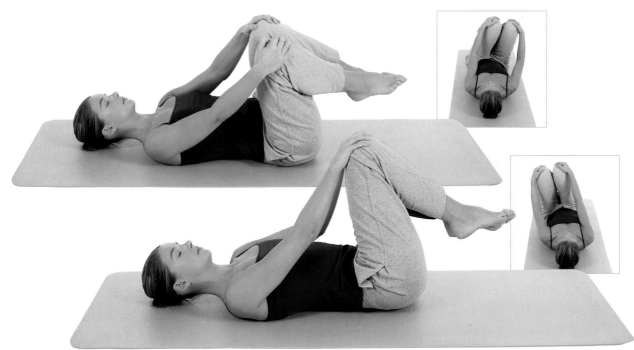

2 circle

• Very slowly and gently, circle both legs from the hips in a clockwise direction and then anti-clockwise 5–10 times each way.

pelvic clocks

This will help you learn pelvic awareness while working your abdominals and freeing the pelvis from tension. Once you are familiar with pelvic clocks you can try them in other positions, for example in a foetal position lying on your side, sitting in a chair, kneeling on all fours or standing with your feet hip width apart.

BENEFITS

Teaches the pelvic awareness required for stability in all Synergize™ Pilates exercises.

- Lie flat on your back, or stand, relaxed, with your legs slightly apart, your arms straight but relaxed, your palms facing your sides.
- Imagine a clock face on your stomach – with your pubic bone at 6 o'clock and your belly button at 12 o'clock. Visualize a pearl sitting in the middle of your belly (the clock face).
- By engaging your pelvic floor 30 per cent, visualize the pearl roll from 6 o'clock to 7 to 8 and so on, right around the clock until you reach 6 o'clock again. Avoid gripping through your thighs and keep your movements small and controlled.
- Try the exercise both anti- and clockwise. You will find some areas of the clock will be easily moved internally while others are tight and more challenging. 5 o'clock and 7 o'clock are commonly tighter than the rest. See where your tensions lie – learn to be aware of them and notice your improvements.

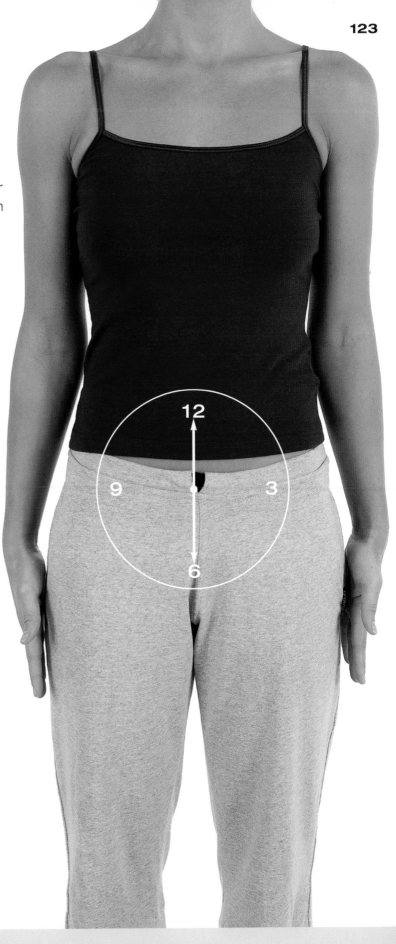

opening and closing the *chi*

This exercise is aimed at improving your health while removing blocked energy from the body during PMT or periods. It is very important that you master the timing of your breath with the physical movement. Take your time with your practice and let your breath be the guide.

BENEFITS
Trains the breath to become easier and more fluid with dynamic movement.

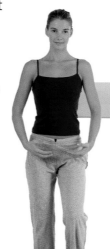

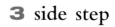

3 side step
• As you inhale deeper, raise your arms further to the sides and step with your left leg out to the side.

2 initiate breathing
• As you inhale, bring your hands close together.

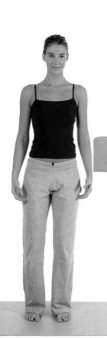

1 soft neutral
• Stand in neutral, relaxed and calm, with your hands by your sides. Your feet should be hip width apart and your shoulders relaxed. Zip in through your abdominals and chest.

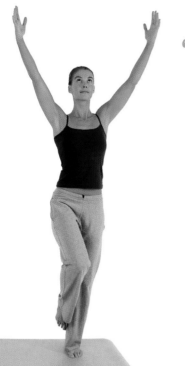

'raise your arms up to the sun gathering all of its energy'

4 open the *chi*

• Keep breathing in and raise your arms up to the sun gathering all of its energy. Keep the left ball of your foot into the floor but keep your heel raised.

6 closure

• Push the energy down towards your pelvis keeping your fingers feathery. Return back to your starting position with both feet flat on the floor.

• Repeat 5–10 times each side and notice how your breathing becomes deeper and more fluid as you practise.

5 close the *chi*

• Start to exhale when your arms meet at the top. Lower your arms down in front of your body, keeping your fingers soft. Stroke the energy as you lower your hands exhaling stagnant *chi*.

immune boosters

side rolls

This will help increase the rotation of the spine with stability of the abdominals for everyday twisting movements. You will also experience more tone in your waist (your abdominal oblique muscles).

BENEFITS
Releases toxins into the breath and out of your body's system.

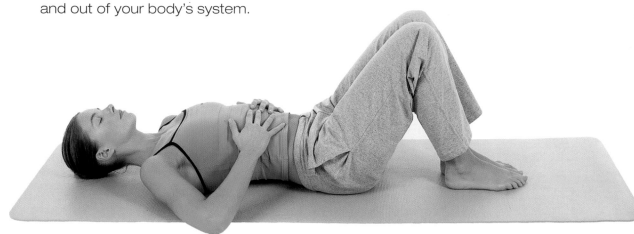

1 neutral semi-supine
• Lie on your back with your legs bent and your feet flat on the floor. Ensure that your spine is in neutral. Place your hands flat on your abdomen.

'If you feel "wound up" by life, enjoy the feeling of unwinding as you come out of the roll.'

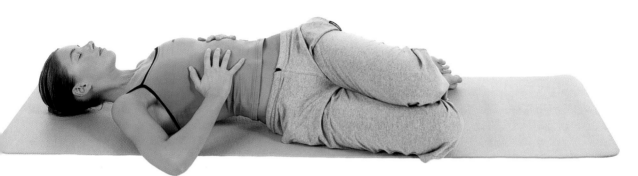

2 roll to right

- Inhale deeply into your lungs and fill them to prepare. Exhale and zip in your abdominals and hollow your belly. Roll your head to your left and your knees to your right.

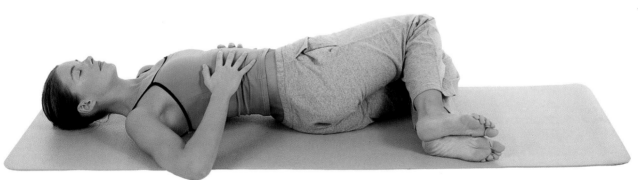

3 roll to left

- Inhale, still zipping, and exhale through your strong core to bring your knees and head back to the centre.
- Exhale and take your head and legs to the other side. Think of rolling each part of your back off the floor in sequence and then returning your rib cage, waist, the small of your back and your buttocks back to the floor.

the hundred

The exercise involves four levels of effort, which you should work through slowly – the level 4 option will take some time to perfect, so take your time. Hold all the positions for 3–5 breaths and repeat 8–12 times.

BENEFITS
Recharges the energy through your core and provides a strong Pilates-based movement to deal with everyday lifting chores and tasks that require core strength.

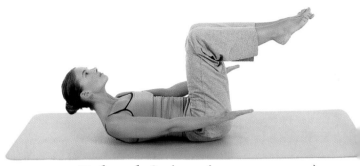

2 level 2 (getting stronger)

- Inhale and prepare your breath by zipping in a little tighter through the waist and spine.
- As you exhale, lift your head and upper torso off the floor to engage your abdominals even further.

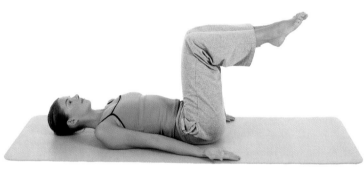

2 level 1 (just starting out)

- Inhale, zip in and prepare your breath. Rotate your hands so your palms face upwards
- Exhale and lift both feet off the floor while staying in neutral alignment. There should be a small space beneath your spine through which a piece of paper could be slid clean to the other side.

1 neutral semi-supine

- Lie on your back with your legs bent and your feet and hands flat on the floor. Ensure neutral alignment by zipping in through the abdominals and lengthening your chest.

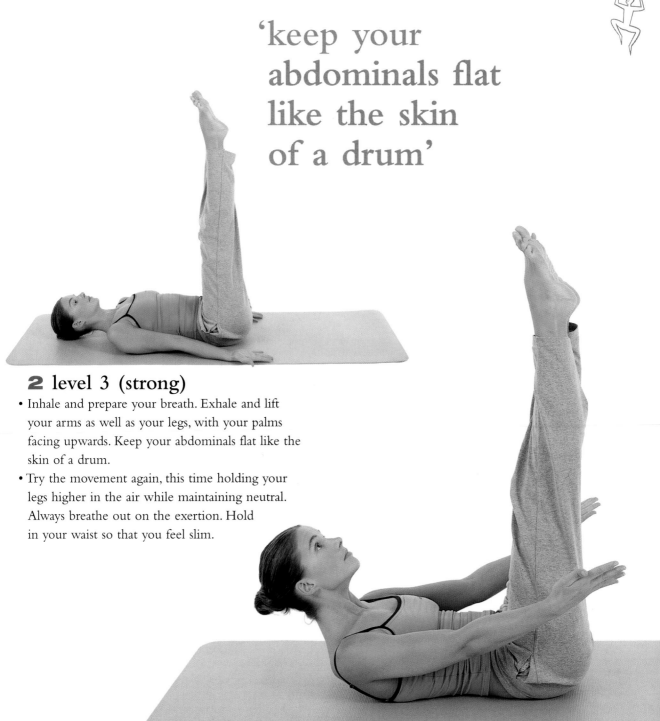

'keep your
abdominals flat
like the skin
of a drum'

2 level 3 (strong)

- Inhale and prepare your breath. Exhale and lift
  your arms as well as your legs, with your palms
  facing upwards. Keep your abdominals flat like the
  skin of a drum.
- Try the movement again, this time holding your
  legs higher in the air while maintaining neutral.
  Always breathe out on the exertion. Hold
  in your waist so that you feel slim.

2 level 4 (advanced)

- Inhale and zip in. Exhale and keep your legs long
  and straight while lifting up your torso and arms
  at the same time. Do not allow the abdominals to
  'dome'. Pull your belly in towards your spine.

lying thigh lengthener

A refreshing stretch that lengthens the tight muscles of the thighs that are heavily used in everyday life.

BENEFITS
Lengthens the thighs and releases tension from these often overused muscles. If you find your thighs thicken easily, this stretch will elongate the muscle fibres and give your thighs a slimmer appearance.

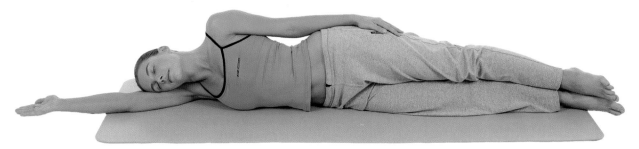

1 left start position

• Lie on your right side with your ankles, knees, hips and shoulders stacked in a straight line.
• Stretch out the supporting arm straight beneath your head for support and balance. Pull your belly in towards your spine.

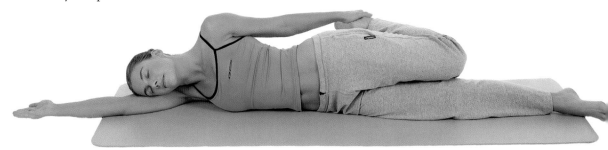

2 left thigh stretch

• Inhale and prepare your breath for the exhalation.
• Exhale and flex your left leg bringing your ankle behind you towards the buttocks. Grasp your ankle and ease into the exhale by bringing the ankle into your bottom. Feel your thigh lengthen.

'feel your thighs lengthen'

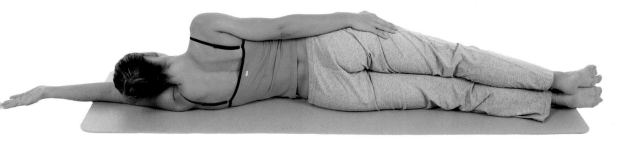

3 right start position
- Roll on to your other side, maintaining your stacked position.
- Stretch out the supporting arm beneath your head for support and balance as before. Pull your belly in towards your spine.

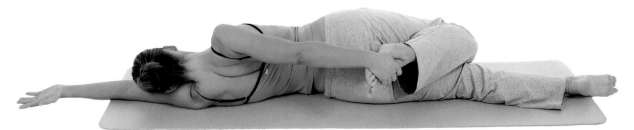

4 right thigh stretch
- Hollow out your belly and ease the right ankle behind you into the buttocks in the same way.
- Repeat 5–10 times, alternating sides.

meridian massage

This massage helps to release stagnant *chi* through the main energy points on the sides of the body.

BENEFITS

Sometimes energy gets blocked in your internal energy channels, just like a kink in a hosepipe. Use this massage to kick start the stagnant *chi* and feel instantly more energized.

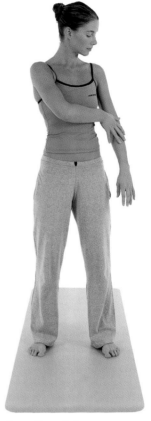

3 back *chi*

• Turn your palm to face behind you and start stroking the energy up the back of the arm, raising the energy towards the upper body.

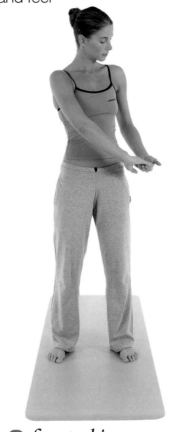

2 front *chi*

• Continue stroking, moving any stagnant *chi* down towards the fingertips and out through each individual finger.

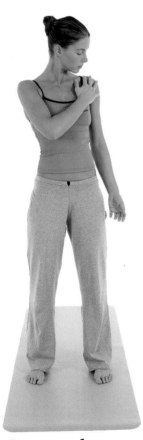

1 neutral

• Stand in wide neutral stance (see page 35). Turn the palm of your left hand to face the front. Using your right hand, stroke with a pushing action down the inside of your left arm.

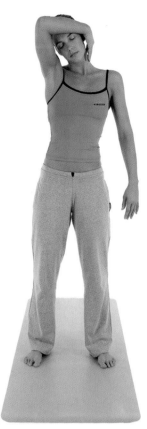

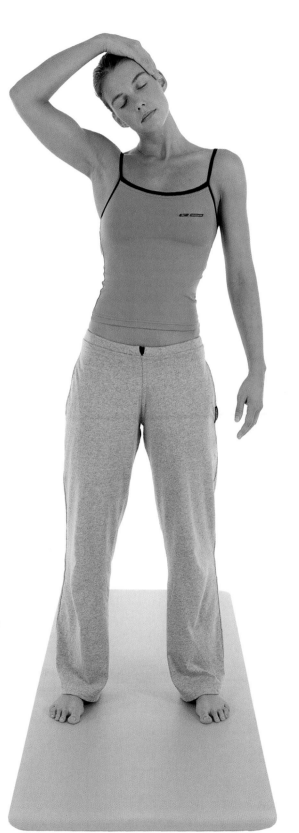

4 neck *chi*

- Continue stroking the energy upwards, all the way along the left shoulder and up through the side of the neck, easing any blockages and moving them on their way.

5 sealing the *chi*

- Continue stroking all the way up to the side of the head. Tilt your head slightly to the side to surrender to the energy exchange.
- Repeat the stroking movements on the other side of your body, and do alternate sides 5–10 times.

the swan

This is a fantastic release for the hip flexors, which can become very tight through long periods of sitting, for example when travelling. This will also help with your hip mobility and the ability to move more smoothly from this area.

BENEFITS
You will move more easily through the hips and your stride will lengthen.

1 preparation stance
- Stand in neutral with your right leg forwards and your left leg back, both feet facing forwards.
- Slowly lower your body to the ground in this split stance position. Bend through the front leg and stretch out the rear leg behind you.
- Ease all the way down through the hip in the front leg until both legs are on the floor. Ensure the right foot is angled across the body and focus on sitting into the hip rather than the knee.

'pull through your abdominals at all times to support and protect you'

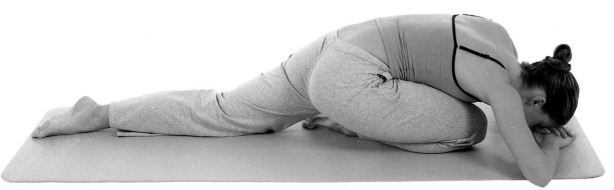

2 swan pose

- Inhale and zip up through the core. Exhale and release your upper torso slowly down over the front right knee. Pull through your abdominals at all times to support and protect you.
- Stay in this position for about 3–5 breaths and ease further into the hip as you exhale each time.

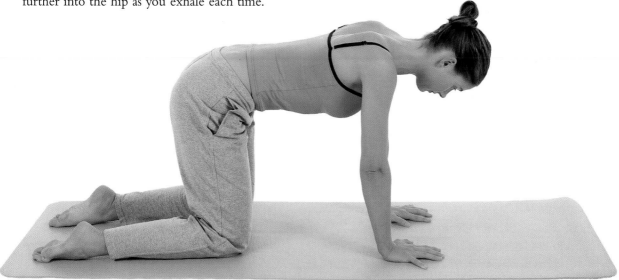

3 swan recovery

- Inhale and slowly elevate your torso back to the box position.
- Exhale. Use your arms to help you push up from the floor and lift your body out of your seated pose. Lengthen up through the legs slowly. Return back to the split stance position.
- Repeat 3 times each side with breaks in between. Work up to 6 times each side as you relax more with the posture.

headache solutions

nodding dog

This releases tension in the muscles at the base of skull and at the rear of the neck. It can prevent headaches if practised in time.

BENEFITS
This loosens any tension in the shoulder muscles, cervical vertebrae (neck), and face.

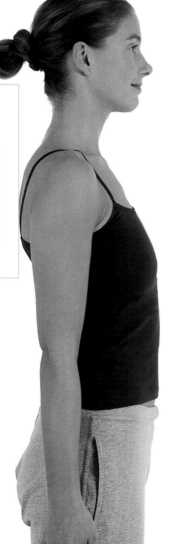

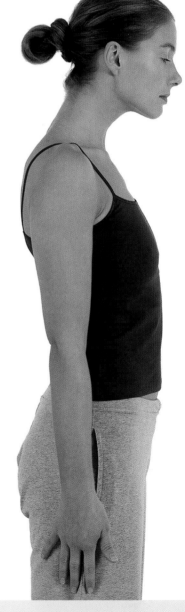

1 nodding dog

• Sit or stand in neutral with your body long and strong and your core zipped up out to the chest. Ensure your head is centred between the shoulder girdle.

• Imagine that your head is balancing on the top of your spine. Be aware of any movement the neck makes to alter this balancing act. Slowly begin to nod your head gently, back and forth like the model nodding dogs seen in the backs of cars. The nods should be hardly noticeable in a mirror.

'Don't take a tablet –
simply spend ten minutes
releasing the tension
felt from a headache.'

2 side dogs

- Now repeat the process but work from side to side.
- Repeat both the front to back and side to side head movements 10–20 times each.

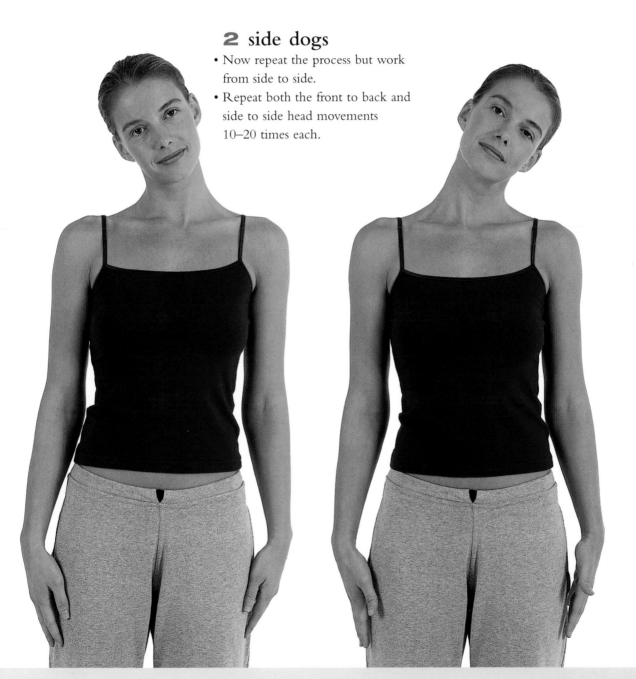

easy twist

This a fantastic movement for releasing the tension within the spine that can sometimes creep up into the neck and build towards a headache.

BENEFITS

Releases spinal tension that may affect the ability to rotate through the back. It also allows the hips to free and the chest to release from tension.

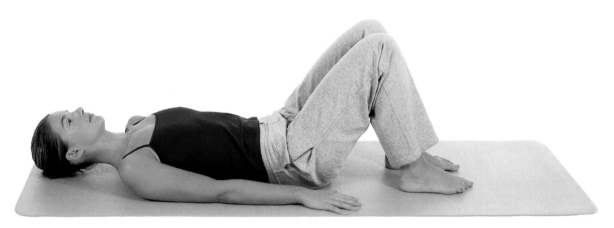

1 neutral semi-supine
• Lie on your back with your legs bent and your feet flat on the floor. Remain in neutral.

'twisting the trunk gives a gentle squeeze to the organs, flushing out deoxygenated blood and allowing fresh blood to enter and nourish the tissues'

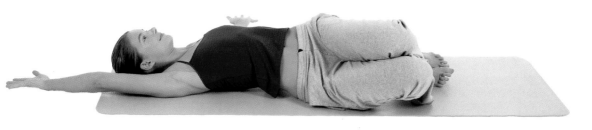

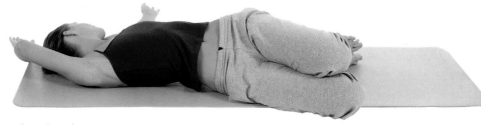

2 flush the twist right

- Inhale and prepare. As you exhale, simultaneously twist your hips and knees to the right and your arms and head over towards the left. Feel a great stretch up the spine and waist areas.

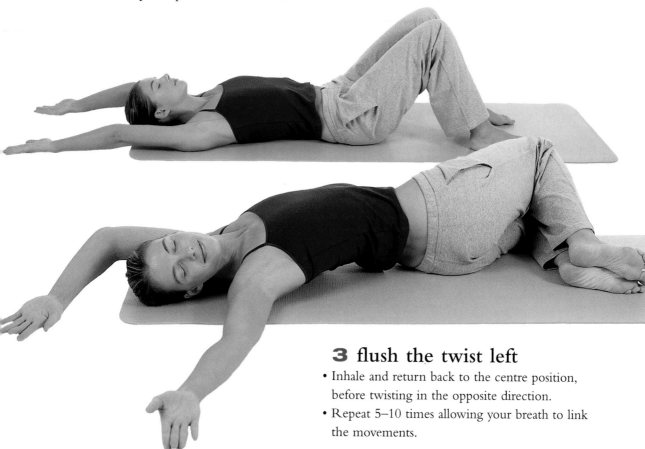

3 flush the twist left

- Inhale and return back to the centre position, before twisting in the opposite direction.
- Repeat 5–10 times allowing your breath to link the movements.

head massage

These are easy to do, yet very effective exercises for easing tension in the cervical (neck) vertebrae and massaging the back of the skull into the floor.

BENEFITS
Releases tension in the neck and allows the jaw to relax aiding relaxation, skin rejuvenation and restful sleep.

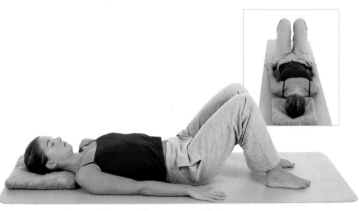

1 relaxation position

• Adopt the Relaxation position with your head on a shallow pillow or towel. Keep your head firmly centred and your neck long.

• Allow your jaw to release and the tongue to widen at its base. Soften your breast bones and allow your shoulder blades to widen and melt into the earth.

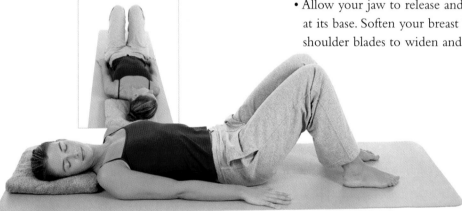

2 head massage roll

• Allow your head to roll slowly to one side.

• Bring it back to the centre and then over to the other side. Do not rush – take your time.

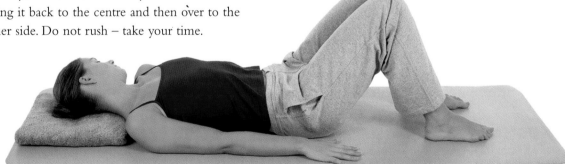

3 deeper head massage tip

• When your neck feels free, bring your head back to the centre and gently tuck in your chin. Imagine you are holding a small kiwi fruit beneath the chin – you do not wish to crush it but just gently hold it.

• Repeat the neck rolling and chin tucking 5–10 times.

facial massage

This exercise will relieve and prevent eyestrain, which in turn can produce headaches if not properly counteracted. It also softens the skin around the eyes reducing fine lines and wrinkles.

BENEFITS
Prevents and relieves eyestrain.

1 start with the eyes

• Begin by pressing your thumbs or middle fingers on the point at the inner end of each eye. Exert as much pressure as possible for about 10 seconds. If you feel pain it indicates that there is tension here.

2 move outwards

• Now move your thumbs or middle fingers out towards the outside of the eye, applying comfortable pressure along the brow.

3 finish at your temples

• Now move your thumbs or middle fingers out towards your temples, applying comfortable pressure.

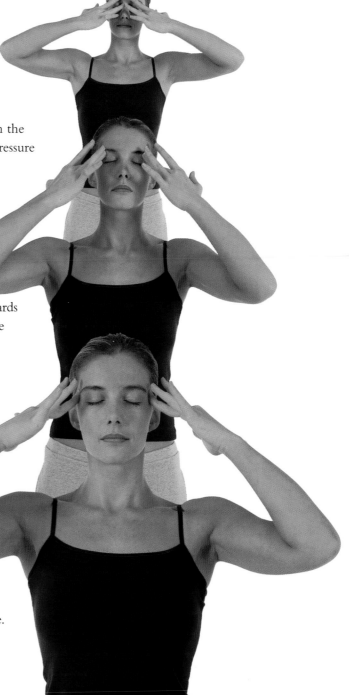

index

acknowledgements

Executive editor Jane McIntosh
Managing editor Clare Churly
Executive art editor Rozelle Bentheim
Designers Maggie Town and Beverly Price
Senior Production Controller Jo Sim
Photography Peter Pugh-Cook
Illustrator Bounford.com